Treatment of Periodontal Disease

Guest Editor

FRANK A. SCANNAPIECO, DMD, PhD

DENTAL CLINICS OF NORTH AMERICA

www.dental.theclinics.com

January 2010 • Volume 54 • Number 1

SAUNDERS an imprint of ELSEVIER, Inc.

W.B. SAUNDERS COMPANY
A Division of Elsevier Inc.

1600 John F. Kennedy Boulevard • Suite 1800 • Philadelphia, Pennsylvania 19103-2899

http://www.dental.theclinics.com

DENTAL CLINICS OF NORTH AMERICA Volume 54, Number 1
January 2010 ISSN 0011-8532, ISBN-13: 978-1-4377-1810-2

Editor: John Vassallo; j.vassallo@elsevier.com
Developmental Editor: Donald Mumford

Dental Clinics of North America (ISSN 0011-8532) is published quarterly by Elsevier Inc., 360 Park Avenue South, New York, NY 10010-1710. Months of issue are January, April, July, and October. Business and Editorial Offices: 1600 John F. Kennedy Boulevard, Suite 1800, Philadelphia, PA 19103-2899. Periodicals postage paid at New York, NY and additional mailing offices. Subscription prices are $224.00 per year (domestic individuals), $382.00 per year (domestic institutions), $108.00 per year (domestic students/residents), $266.00 per year (Canadian individuals), $481.00 per year (Canadian institutions), $321.00 per year (international individuals), $481.00 per year (international institutions), and $162.00 per year (international and Canadian students/residents). International air speed delivery is included in all *Clinics* subscription prices. All prices are subject to change without notice. **POSTMASTER:** Send address changes to *Dental Clinics of North America*, Elsevier Health Sciences Division, Subscription Customer Service, 3251 Riverport Lane, Maryland Heights, MO 63043. **Customer Service (orders, claims, online, change of address): Elsevier Health Sciences Division, Subscription Customer Service, 3251 Riverport Lane, Maryland Heights, MO 63043. Tel: 1-800-654-2452 (U.S. and Canada). Fax: 314-447-8029. E-mail: journalscustomerservice-usa@elsevier.com (for print support); journalsonlinesupport-usa@elsevier.com (for online support).**

Reprints. For copies of 100 or more, of articles in this publication, please contact the Commercial Reprints Department, Elsevier Inc., 360 Park Avenue South, New York, NY 10010-1710. Tel.: 212-633-3812; Fax: 212-462-1935; E-mail: reprints@elsevier.com.

The Dental Clinics of North America is covered in *MEDLINE/PubMed (Index Medicus)*, *Current Contents/Clinical Medicine*, *ISI/BIOMED* and *Clinahl*.

Printed and bound by CPI Group (UK) Ltd, Croydon, CR0 4YY

Transferred to Digital Print 2011

Contributors

GUEST EDITOR

FRANK A. SCANNAPIECO, DMD, PhD
Professor and Chair, Department of Oral Biology, University at Buffalo, The State
University of New York, School of Dental Medicine, Buffalo, New York

AUTHORS

MARY ELIZABETH AICHELMANN-REIDY, DDS
Associate Professor, Department of Periodontics, Associate Director, Postgraduate
Program in Periodontics, Dental School, University of Maryland, Baltimore, Maryland

SEBASTIANO ANDREANA, DDS, MS
Associate Professor, Director of Implant Dentistry, Department of Restorative Dentistry,
University at Buffalo, School of Dental Medicine, Buffalo, New York

DANAE A. APATZIDOU, DDS, PhD
Teaching Associate, Dental School, Department of Preventive Dentistry, Periodontology
and Biology of Implants, Aristotle University of Thessaloniki, Thessaloniki, Greece

HALA BADAWI, DDS
Dental Resident, Marquette University, School of Dentistry, Milwaukee, Wisconsin

GRISHONDRA L. BRANCH-MAYS, DDS, MS
Associate Professor, Department of Periodontics, Director, Predoctoral Education in
Periodontics, Dental School, University of Maryland, Baltimore, Maryland

JOHN CAVALLARO Jr, DDS
Clinical Associate Professor, Department of Periodontology & Implant Dentistry, New York
University College of Dentistry, Freehold, New Jersey; Private Practice, Brooklyn,
New York

NOK CHHUN, MS, MPH
Research Scientist, Graduate Program in Clinical Research, Department of Epidemiology,
New York University College of Dentistry, New York, New York

CHARLES M. COBB, DDS, MS, PhD
Professor Emeritus, Department of Periodontics, School of Dentistry, University of
Missouri-Kansas City, Kansas City, Missouri

DAVID L. COCHRAN, DDS, MS, PhD, MMSc
Chair and Associate Professor, Department of Periodontics, The University of Texas,
Health Science Center at San Antonio, San Antonio, Texas

DONALD J. COLUZZI, DDS
Associate Professor, Department of Preventive and Restorative Dental Sciences,
University of California San Francisco School of Dentistry, San Francisco, California

ANANDA P. DASANAYAKE, BDS, MPH, PhD, FACE
Professor and Director, Graduate Program in Clinical Research, New York University
College of Dentistry, New York, New York

ANDREW R. DENTINO, DDS, PhD
Professor and Undergraduate Program Director, Department of Surgical Sciences, Marquette University, School of Dentistry, Milwaukee, Wisconsin

GARY GREENSTEIN, DDS, MS
Clinical Professor, Department of Periodontology & Implant Dentistry, New York University College of Dentistry; Private Practice, Freehold, New Jersey

GIUSEPPE INTINI, DDS, PhD
Department of Developmental Biology, Harvard School of Dental Medicine, Boston, Massachusetts

MOAWIA M. KASSAB, DDS, MS
Assistant Professor, Department of Surgical Sciences, Marquette University, School of Dentistry, Milwaukee, Wisconsin

DENIS F. KINANE, BDS, FDSRCS, FDSRCPS, PhD
Professor of Periodontology and Professor of Pathology, University of Pennsylvania School of Denstistry, School of Dental Medicine, Philadelphia, Pennsylvania; Associate Dean for Research, School of Dentistry, University of Louisville, Louisville, Kentucky

KEITH L. KIRKWOOD, DDS, PhD
Department of Craniofacial Biology, College of Dental Medicine; Center for Oral Health Research, Medical University of South Carolina, Charleston, South Carolina

JOE W. KRAYER, DDS, MS
Department of Stomatology, College of Dental Medicine, Medical University of South Carolina, Charleston, South Carolina

JAEBUM LEE, DDS, MSc, PhD
Chief Clinical Scientist, Laboratory for Applied Periodontal & Craniofacial Regeneration (LAPCR), Department of Periodontics and Oral Biology, Medical College of Georgia School of Dentistry, Augusta, Georgia

RENATA S. LEITE, DMD, MS
Department of Stomatology, College of Dental Medicine; Center for Oral Health Research, Medical University of South Carolina, Charleston, South Carolina

SAMUEL B. LOW, DDS, MS
Professor, Department of Periodontics, College of Dentistry, University of Florida, Gainesville, Florida

MARK A. REYNOLDS, DDS, PhD
Professor and Chair, Department of Periodontics, Director, Postgraduate Program in Periodontics, Dental School, University of Maryland, Baltimore, Maryland

FRANK A. SCANNAPIECO, DMD, PhD
Professor and Chair, Department of Oral Biology, University at Buffalo, The State University of New York, School of Dental Medicine, Buffalo, New York

ANDREAS STAVROPOULOS, DDS, PhD
Associate Professor, Department of Periodontology, University of Aarhus School of Dentistry, Aarhus C, Denmark

CRISTIANO SUSIN, DDS, MSD, PhD
Senior Scientist, Laboratory for Applied Periodontal & Craniofacial Regeneration (LAPCR), Department of Periodontics and Oral Biology, Medical College of Georgia School of Dentistry, Augusta, Georgia

DENNIS TARNOW, DDS
Professor and Chairman, Department of Periodontology & Implant Dentistry, New York University College of Dentistry, Freehold, New Jersey; Private Practice, New York, New York

CRISTINA C. VILLAR, DDS, MS, PhD
Assistant Professor, Department of Periodontics, The University of Texas, Health Science Center at San Antonio, San Antonio, Texas

ULF M.E. WIKESJÖ, DDS, DMD, PhD
Professor, Director, Laboratory for Applied Periodontal & Craniofacial Regeneration (LAPCR), Department of Periodontics and Oral Biology, Medical College of Georgia School of Dentistry, Augusta, Georgia

Contents

The comparison of the efficacy of surgical and nonsurgical procedures revealed that scaling and root planing alone or in combination with flap procedures are effective methods for the treatment of chronic periodontitis. Also, the consistent message is that in treating deep pockets, open-flap debridement results in greater probing pocket depth reduction and clinical attachment gain than nonsurgical modalities. Nonsurgical modalities in shallower pockets consistently involve less post-therapy recession and are clearly recognized as being more conservative. Research is still needed on the clinical benefit of the granulation tissue removal that is a feature of periodontal surgical therapy and, to a lesser extent, occurs through indirect trauma in nonsurgical therapy.

Periodontal diseases are initiated by subgingival periodontal pathogens in susceptible periodontal sites. The host immune response toward periodontal pathogens helps to sustain periodontal disease and eventual alveolar bone loss. Numerous adjunctive therapeutic strategies have evolved to manage periodontal diseases. Systemic and local antibiotics, antiseptics, and past and future host immune modulatory agents are reviewed and discussed to facilitate the dental practitioner's appreciation of this ever-growing field in clinical periodontics.

For many intraoral soft-tissue surgical procedures the laser has become a desirable and dependable alternative to traditional scalpel surgery. However, the use of dental lasers in periodontal therapy is controversial. This article presents the current peer-reviewed evidence on the use of dental lasers for the treatment of chronic periodontitis.

Bone replacement grafts are widely used to promote bone formation and periodontal regeneration. Conventional surgical approaches, such as open flap debridement, provide critical access to evaluate and detoxify root surfaces as well as establish improved periodontal form and architecture; however, these surgical techniques offer only limited potential in restoring or reconstituting component periodontal tissues. A wide range of bone grafting materials, including bone grafts and bone graft substitutes, have been applied and evaluated clinically, including autografts, allografts, xenografts, and alloplasts (synthetic/semisynthetic materials). This review provides an overview of the biologic function and clinical application of bone replacement grafts for periodontal regeneration. Emphasis is placed on the clinical and biologic goals of periodontal regeneration as well as evidence-based treatment outcomes.

The concept that only fibroblasts from the periodontal ligament or undifferentiated mesenchymal cells have the potential to re-create the original periodontal attachment has been long recognized. Based on this concept, guided tissue regeneration has been applied with variable success to regenerate periodontal defects. Quantitative analysis of clinical outcomes after guided tissue regeneration suggests that this therapy is a successful and predictable procedure to treat narrow intrabony defects and class II mandibular furcations, but offers limited benefits in the treatment of other types of periodontal defects.

Several growth and differentiation factors have shown potential as therapeutic agents to support periodontal wound healing/regeneration, although optimal dosage, release kinetics, and suitable delivery systems are still unknown. Experimental variables, including delivery systems, dose, and the common use of poorly characterized preclinical models, make it difficult to discern the genuine efficacy of each of these factors. Only a few growth and differentiation factors have reached clinical evaluation. It appears that well-defined discriminating preclinical models followed by well-designed clinical trials are needed to further investigate the true potential of these and other candidate factors. Thus, current research is focused on finding relevant growth and differentiation factors, optimal dosages, and the best approaches for delivery to develop clinically meaningful therapies in patient-centered settings.

The principal reason for providing periodontal therapy is to achieve periodontal health and retain the dentition. Patients with a history of periodontitis represent a unique group of individuals who previously succumbed to a bacterial challenge. Therefore, it is important to address the management and survival rate of implants in these patients. Systematic reviews often are cited in this article, because they provide a high level of evidence and facilitate reviewing a vast amount of information in a succinct manner.

Treatment of Gingival Recession   129

Moawia M. Kassab, Hala Badawi, and Andrew R. Dentino

Gingival recession is an intriguing and complex phenomenon. Recession frequently disturbs patients because of sensitivity and esthetics. Many surgical techniques have been introduced to treat gingival recession, including those involving autogenous tissue grafting, various flap designs, orthodontics, and guided tissue regeneration. This article describes different clinical approaches to treat gingival recession with emphasis on techniques that show promising results and root coverage.

Future Approaches in Periodontal Regeneration: Gene Therapy, Stem Cells, and RNA Interference   141

Giuseppe Intini

Periodontal disease is a major public health issue and the development of effective therapies to treat the disease and regenerate periodontal tissue is an important goal of today's medicine. This article highlights recent scientific advancements in gene therapy, stem cell biology, and RNA interference with the intent of identifying their potential in periodontal tissue regeneration. Results from basic research, preclinical, and clinical studies indicate that these fields of research may soon contribute to more effective regenerative therapies for periodontal disease.

Restorative Options for the Periodontal Patient   157

Sebastiano Andreana

Periodontal and restorative dentistry are mutually important facets of clinical dentistry. Today's clinicians have many treatment options at their disposal, including biotolerant restorative materials and implants, to maintain periodontal health. It is crucial for the clinician to understand the biologic principles that form the foundation for restorative reconstruction of the periodontally involved tooth. This article discusses new techniques and trends in the critical management of the restorations, particularly at the gingival margins, and explores the role of implant dentistry as an option for the restorative plan of the periodontal patient.

"Does Periodontal Therapy Reduce the Risk for Systemic Diseases?"   163

Frank A. Scannapieco, Ananda P. Dasanayake, and Nok Chhun

Periodontal disease is treated by various approaches, including simple oral hygiene practices, professional mechanical debridement, antimicrobial therapy and periodontal surgery. There is evidence to associate periodontal disease with several systemic diseases and conditions, including myocardial infarction, adverse pregnancy outcomes, diabetes mellitus, and respiratory disease. This article reviews the published literature that describes the effects of periodontal treatment on cardiovascular diseases, adverse pregnancy outcomes, diabetes mellitus, and respiratory disease. While some progress has been made, further research is required to understand the value of periodontal interventions in the prevention of systemic diseases.

Index   183

FORTHCOMING ISSUES

April 2010
Endodontics
Frederic Barnett, DMD
Guest Editor

July 2010
Current Concepts in Cariology
Douglas A. Young, DDS, MS, MBA
Margherita Fontana, DDS, PhD
and Mark S. Wolff, DDS, PhD
Guest Editors

October 2010
Updates in Dental Anesthesia and Analgesia
Paul A. Moore, DMD, PhD, MPH
Elliot V. Hersh, DMD, PhD and
Sean G. Boynes, DMD, MS
Guest Editors

RECENT ISSUES

October 2009
Orofacial Trauma and Emergency Care
Sami M.A. Chogle, BDS, DMD, MSD
and Gerald A. Ferretti, DDS, MS, MPH
Guest Editors

July 2009
Oral Health Care Access
Gary A. Colangelo, DDS, MGA
Guest Editor

April 2009
The Special Care Patient
Burton S. Wasserman, DDS, DABSCD
Guest Editor

RELATED INTEREST

Oral and Maxillofacial Surgery Clinics of North America February 2007 (Vol. 19, No. 1)
Management of Impacted Teeth
Vincent J. Perciaccante, DDS, *Guest Editor*

THE CLINICS ARE NOW AVAILABLE ONLINE!

Access your subscription at:
www.theclinics.com

Preface

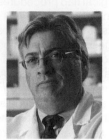

Frank A. Scannapieco, DMD, PhD
Guest Editor

Until the middle of the twentieth century, the treatment of periodontal diseases was based on inferences on the cause of the disease from the study of histologic material and expert opinion. Thus, at that time, such investigators as Shluger[1] called for the need for the therapist to eliminate the periodontal pocket, create harmonious gingival form, and recontour the osseous architecture to prevent progression or recurrence of periodontal pocketing. Preservation of "physiologic architecture," elimination of food traps, and maintenance of a wide zone of keratinized gingiva were all desired end points of periodontal therapy. Thus, much attention was paid to correction of anatomic deformities to enable the patient to adequately perform oral hygiene.

Starting in the late 1950s, scientific studies began to identify the major etiologic factors that cause periodontal disease (the microorganisms of dental plaque) and the modifying risk factors (eg, smoking, age, gender, underlying systemic diseases). Well-designed clinical trials compared nonsurgical therapy (scaling and root planing) to surgical procedures and assessed outcomes, such as pocket depths and attachment levels.[2–6] These studies showed that, for most patients, thorough debridement of the teeth (ie, removal of all supragingival and subgingival microbial deposits) often was as effective as periodontal surgery to prevent progression of alveolar bone loss in patients with chronic periodontitis. Restoration of tissues lost to disease was not an expected outcome.

Today, efforts continue to focus on preventing periodontal attachment loss from starting or progressing. In addition, however, the search is on to devise therapies to regenerate lost tissue. Periodontal researchers are seeking ways to apply the newly developed technologies (eg, lasers, gene therapy, growth factors, drug delivery systems, implants) to restore lost tissue and function. Therefore, one goal of the present issue is to present a comprehensive picture on the state-of-the-science of periodontal treatment.

Another goal is to systematically present a state-of-the-art summary of the full range of treatment options available to the dental practitioner to prevent and manage periodontal diseases. Every effort was made by each author to articulate the strength of the evidence supporting the use of each approach.

Dent Clin N Am 54 (2010) xi–xiii
doi:10.1016/j.cden.2009.10.003
0011-8532/09/$ – see front matter © 2010 Elsevier Inc. All rights reserved.

dental.theclinics.com

The issue begins with a discussion of nonsurgical periodontal therapy, now a main-stay of conventional practice. Apatzidou and Kinane explain that both scaling and root planing alone and scaling and root planing combined with surgical flap procedures are effective in treating chronic periodontitis in terms of achieving attachment level gain and reducing gingival inflammation. They review results from the studies of Quirynen and colleagues,[7] who advocate the use of one-stage full-mouth disinfection (scaling and root planing all teeth completed over two sessions within 24 hours with the use of chlorhexidine for mouth rinsing and disinfection of all intraoral niches). Apat-zidou and Kinane also discuss efficacy of ultrasonic instrumentation compared with conventional manual instrumentation. It is clear that, regardless of approach, disrup-tion and removal of the microbial biofilm and the initiation and establishment of metic-ulous plaque control constitute the key elements of successful nonsurgical periodontal treatment.

Krayer and colleagues review the use of antibiotics, antiseptics, anti-inflammatory agents, and other host modulatory agents in periodontal therapy. It seems evident from this review that all pharmaceutical approaches available to date should be used not as stand-alone interventions, but to augment mechanical therapy to treat periodontal disease.

One technology that seems to fascinate both dental professionals and the public is the medical laser. Cobb and colleagues' review of the literature argues that the use of the laser to treat periodontal diseases does not achieve results that exceed those of present standards of care. Furthermore, many questions remain to be answered regarding the use of lasers as a singular modality or as an adjunct for the treatment of periodontitis.

Periodontists have long hoped to identify procedures to predictably regenerate lost periodontal tissues. Thus, several reviews that summarize the strengths and weak-nesses of growth factors, guided tissue regeneration, and bone grafts are all covered herein. Further information on future approaches that may be in use for periodontal regeneration, such as gene therapy, RNA interference, and stem cells, are also re-viewed. RNA-based therapeutics, such as RNA interference, and other approaches for tissue regeneration are still in their infancy. While not yet available for clinical appli-cations, such theoretical approaches offer exciting prospects for future strategies to regain the tissues lost to the ravages of periodontal inflammation.

A welcome addition to the dentist's armamentarium is the dental implant. This rapidly improving technology adds an important option for the replacement of lost teeth. While osseointegration of dental implants is a predictable treatment modality, the placement of implants in the periodontal patient presents a unique situation for the dental practitioner. Greenstein and colleagues' comprehensive review on the use of implants in the periodontal patient should help the dentist decide whether to attempt to treat the periodontally involved tooth or extract it in favor of implant placement.

A clinical situation sometimes challenging to treat is gingival recession. This condition must be corrected should it cause patient discomfort or affect esthetics. Kassab and colleagues provide a comprehensive review of the indications for correc-tion of recessions, as well as a variety of techniques presently available for this purpose.

A growing literature suggests that periodontal inflammation and infection may have serious ramifications for systemic health. If true, it is possible that prevention or treat-ment of periodontal disease could reduce the risk for such systemic conditions as cardiovascular disease and stroke, adverse pregnancy outcomes, diabetes mellitus, and respiratory diseases, such as pneumonia. Thus, an effort is made here to review pertinent clinical trials that have attempted to determine how periodontal therapy affects these systemic conditions.

Finally, it is clear that periodontal treatment certainly affects restorative treatment planning. Andreana addresses issues pertinent to considerations affecting restorative treatment.

It is my pleasure to thank all of the experts who generously gave their time and talents to provide such detailed and well-written articles that make up this issue. It is our hope that this work will inform the modern evidence-based dental practitioner with the background necessary to manage periodontal diseases.

Frank A. Scannapieco, DMD, PhD
Department of Oral Biology
University at Buffalo
The State University of New York
School of Dental Medicine
3435 Main Street
Buffalo, NY 14214, USA

E-mail address:
fas1@buffalo.edu

REFERENCES

1. Shluger S. Osseous resection—a basic principle in periodontal surgery. Oral Surg 1949;70:316–25.
2. Badersten A, Nilveus R, Egelberg J. Effect of nonsurgical periodontal therapy. I. Moderately advanced periodontitis. J Clin Periodontol 1981;8(1):57–72.
3. Renvert S, Badersten A, Nilveus R, et al. Healing after treatment of periodontal intraosseous defects. I. Comparative study of clinical methods. J Clin Periodontol 1981;8(5):387–99.
4. Badersten A, Nilveus R, Egelberg J. Effect of nonsurgical periodontal therapy. III. Single versus repeated instrumentation. J Clin Periodontol 1984;11(2):114–24.
5. Badersten A, Nilveus R, Egelberg J. Effect of nonsurgical periodontal therapy. II. Severely advanced periodontitis. J Clin Periodontol 1984;11(1):63–76.
6. Ramfjord SP, Caffesse RG, Morrison EC, et al. Four modalities of periodontal treatment compared over five years. J Periodont Res 1987;22(3):222–3.
7. Quirynen M, De Soete M, Boschmans G, et al. Benefit of "one-stage full-mouth disinfection" is explained by disinfection and root planing within 24 hours: a randomized controlled trial. J Clin Periodontol 2006;33(9):639–47.

Nonsurgical Mechanical Treatment Strategies for Periodontal Disease

Danae A. Apatzidou, DDS, PhD[a],*,
Denis F. Kinane, BDS, FDSRCS, FDSRCPS, PhD[b,c]

KEYWORDS

- Full-mouth treatment • Root planing • Ultrasonic debridement
- Periodontal pathogens • Host response

EFFICACY OF SCALING AND ROOT PLANING

Numerous investigations support the efficacy of scaling and root planing in the treatment of periodontal disease.[1–4] Typically studies show that posttreatment pocket depth reduction is directly related to the initial pocket depth, with the greatest reduction noted for the deepest pockets.[5–7] A consistent relationship is also found between changes in the attachment levels and initial pocket depth. In a thorough review of the literature, the mean probing pocket reduction and mean attachment gain following scaling and root planing were determined for shallow, deep, and moderately deep sites.[8] Shallow pockets (1–4 mm) and moderately deep sites (4–7 mm) had a mean pocket reduction of 0.03 mm and 1.29 mm, respectively, whereas deep sites (>6 mm) showed the greatest pocket depth reduction of 2.16 mm. The mean attachment gain for shallow, moderately deep, and deep sites was –0.34 mm, 0.55 mm, and 1.19 mm, respectively. This study also showed a mean reduction in bleeding on probing of 57% post-therapy.

Thus, the data highlight the magnitude of the effects of nonsurgical mechanical therapy on periodontal clinical indices and also demonstrate that attachment loss is to be expected when shallow periodontal pockets are scaled and root planed.

EFFICACY OF PERIODONTAL SURGERY

Most of the longitudinal studies demonstrate that scaling and root planing and surgical approaches are similarly effective.[5,6,9–13] Meta-analyses by Antczak-Bouckoms and

[a] Dental School, Department of Preventive Dentistry, Periodontology and Biology of Implants, Aristotle University of Thessaloniki, University Campus, 54124 Greece
[b] Periodontology and Pathology, University of Pennsylvania School of Dentistry, School of Dental Medicine, 240 South 40th Street, Philadelphia, PA 19104-6030, USA
[c] School of Dentistry, University of Louisville, Louisville, KY 40202, USA
* Corresponding author.
E-mail address: perioapatzidou@yahoo.gr (D.A. Apatzidou).

Dent Clin N Am 54 (2010) 1–12
doi:10.1016/j.cden.2009.08.006
0011-8532/09/$ – see front matter © 2010 Elsevier Inc. All rights reserved.
dental.theclinics.com

colleagues,[14] Berkley and colleagues,[15] and Heitz-Mayfield and colleagues[16] evaluated reduction in probing pocket depth (PPD) and gain in clinical attachment levels as primary outcome measures. The reviews are highly consistent in that scaling and root planing alone and scaling and root planing combined with flap procedure are accepted as effective methods for the treatment of chronic periodontitis in attachment level gain and gingival inflammation reduction.

Heitz-Mayfield and co-workers concluded that sites with initial PPD of 1 to 3 mm treated with open flap debridement resulted in significantly greater loss in clinical attachment levels compared with scaling and root planing.[16] When sites with initial PPD of 4 to 6 mm were treated with open flap debridement, there was significantly less clinical attachment level (CAL) gain compared with scaling and root planing. The PPD reduction was significantly greater following the open flap debridement procedure. Finally, when sites with initial PPD greater than 6 mm were treated with surgical procedures, there was significantly more CAL gain than with the standard procedures of scaling and root planing. Open flap debridement resulted in significantly more PPD reduction than did the nonsurgical scaling and root planing approach in these deep pockets.

Lindhe and colleagues[17] demonstrated that in a well-controlled oral hygiene regime, thorough scaling and root planing was equally effective when used alone or in combination with the modified Widman procedure in the treatment of advanced periodontitis. A high frequency of probing depths less than 4 mm was noted following both treatment modalities, and the investigators speculated that the attachment gain after treatment reflected a reduction in the degree of gingival inflammation rather than a true gain of connective tissue attachment. The clinical improvements after mechanical debridement remained unchanged during an 18-month maintenance period. During this period, recurrence occurred, but it was a rare finding and when it did develop it was related to either ineffective prophylactic measures or inadequate debridement during active treatment.[18]

ADVANCES IN NONSURGICAL TREATMENT PROTOCOLS

Quirynen and colleagues[19] introduced the one-stage full-mouth disinfection, including adjunctive use of chlorhexidine (mouth rinsing and disinfection of all intraoral niches), and they compared the clinical and microbiological effects of this treatment strategy with the more traditional treatment of quadrant scaling and root planing at 2-weekly intervals with no adjunctive use of chlorhexidine. The one-stage protocol included full-mouth scaling and root planing under local anesthesia using hand and ultrasonic instruments, completed over 2 sessions within 24 hours. Time spent for treating one quadrant was approximately 1 hour. The disinfection of the oral cavity also involved an extensive application of chlorhexidine to all intraoral niches, such as periodontal pockets, tongue dorsum, tonsils, and oral mucous membranes, chairside and at home, for 2 months. The rationale behind the full-mouth disinfection was to prevent reinfection of the instrumented sites from the remaining untreated pockets and from other intraoral niches.

Thereafter, the Leuven research group conducted a series of clinical trials and consistently demonstrated a superior clinical outcome for the one-stage full-mouth disinfection treatment modality.[19–24] This treatment strategy evolved such that the clinical protocol of the full-mouth scaling and root planing was completed in 24 hours or less, with no adjunctive use of antiseptic agents. However, these reported gains in clinical and microbiological indices achieved for the full-mouth approach by the Leuven group have not been found by subsequent researchers,[25,26] which has generated an ongoing debate as to whether the full-mouth clinical protocol should be the treatment of choice.

Data from other studies provide concurrence that chlorhexidine does not augment the beneficial outcome of periodontal therapy,[27–30] and when this does occur, it is a transient phenomenon rather than a long-term effect.[31,32] However, it should be stressed that in the quoted studies, chlorhexidine was used as a single measure of disinfection in contrast to the treatment protocol of multiple chlorhexidine applications used in the Leuven studies.[19–24] Nevertheless, there is a general agreement in the literature that clinical trials with a lack of meticulous plaque control gave misleadingly promising results for the adjunctive use of chlorhexidine.

A later study by the Leuven research group[24] examined patients with moderately advanced periodontitis and concluded that the benefits of the full-mouth treatment protocol were partially due to the antiseptics and partially, the shorter time for completion of the therapy; this conclusion contradicts earlier findings[23] that questioned the role of the antiseptics in this treatment strategy. The earlier study demonstrated that the full-mouth treatment with chlorhexidine was superior to all other treatment strategies in patients with advanced periodontitis.[23] Although the full-mouth group showed greater improvements in pocket depths and attachment levels compared with the quadrantwise treated group, with antiseptics used in neither group, this failed to reach statistical significance at 8 months ($P \leq .10$). The group that received the quadrantwise treatment in this study[24] scored considerably better in pocket depth reductions than in the earlier study,[23] and this discrepancy may explain the differences in the 2 studies from the same research group.

Apatzidou and Kinane[25] randomized 40 patients into 2 treatment groups (one-day full-mouth root planing versus quadrantwise root planing) and followed these subjects over 6 months. Although the one-day group was mechanically treated on the same day, they were still seen every second week to receive the same amount of oral hygiene instruction and motivation as the quadrantwise group. This resulted in similar plaque indices between the treatment groups throughout the study; this result disagrees with the findings of Vandekerckhove and colleagues,[20] who showed higher plaque indices for the one-stage full-mouth disinfection group after the first month, possibly due to lack of frequent sessions of oral hygiene reinforcement. Periodontitis is a chronic multifactorial inflammatory disease process, which requires the commitment of the patient and the therapist in achieving long-term periodontal stability. Although the full-mouth treatment is completed within hours, patients with periodontitis, especially advanced cases, should be monitored closely and frequently by the therapist until the time of the initial reassessment to optimize the oral hygiene, establish a relationship between patient and therapist, and consolidate the long-term commitment.[33] Considering this argument and in contrast to the conclusions of the Leuven group, full-mouth scaling and root planing, which requires approximately 1 hour of instrumentation per quadrant completed in 1 day or on 2 consecutive days, offers no additional economic advantages over the classic quadrantwise treatment.[34] On the other hand, recent studies point out that single-visit, full-mouth or quadrantwise ultrasonic debridement with or without the adjunctive use of antiseptics is less laborious and time-consuming, yet equally efficacious clinically as the standard periodontal therapy of scaling and root planing.[35,36] Koshy and colleagues[35] reanalyzed the effects of full-mouth and quadrantwise treatment by using ultrasonics rather than hand instrumentation. Their protocol, briefly stated, was to complete full-mouth ultrasonic debridement in 2.5 hours or less with either povidone-iodine or water as irrigant for the ultrasonic device and to compare the clinical outcome and polymerase chain reaction findings of this treatment with the quadrantwise ultrasonic debridement. Their results demonstrated that the single-visit debridement had limited additional benefits over the partial treatment, except that, from a practical perspective, less time was required overall to complete treatment in one visit than over 4 consecutive sessions.

Wennström and co-workers[36] reduced the time frame of periodontal therapy of patients with moderately advanced chronic periodontitis to 1 hour with the use of ultrasonics solely under local anesthesia, if requested by the patient. The reported data demonstrated that the 1-hour treatment resulted in a smaller percentage of "closed" pockets (PPD <5 mm) compared with the classical treatment of quadrant-by-quadrant scaling and root planing with hand instruments on a weekly basis, but it also demonstrated that the efficiency of the initial treatment phase (baseline to 2 months), defined as the time spent for instrumentation divided by the number of closed pockets, was significantly higher for the full-mouth ultrasonic debridement. In this study, oral hygiene instructions were given on 3 occasions in a similar manner for both treatment groups. The investigators highlighted the practical benefits of this treatment approach over the quadrantwise or full-mouth treatment of scaling and root planing, which is either performed over 2 sessions within 24 hours or over 4 sessions at biweekly intervals. Their results suggest that the 1-hour debridement may be a justifiable initial treatment approach for the patient with chronic periodontitis, and they emphasize that fewer appointments and less chair time are required for this treatment that has less postoperative discomfort compared with the traditional approach of quadrant scaling and root planing.

RATIONALE FOR ULTRASONIC DEBRIDEMENT

There has been extensive discussion on whether power-driven devices/ultrasonics are as effective as hand instruments in debriding the root surface. Randomized controlled clinical trials[1,2,37,38] confirmed by other studies[39–42] showed no significant differences between power-driven and hand instrumentation in nonsurgical periodontal treatment. The systematic review by Walmsley and colleagues[43] essentially reiterates that power-driven and conventional hand instrumentation techniques are equally efficacious, and despite extensive research and refinement in the power-driven field, showing substantial clinical improvements with these new methodologies is still some way off. Promising future developments in tip designs and in the generators used to develop power may provide clinical superiority; however, clinical verification of the utility of these advances is still needed. Advantages associated with power-driven instruments include better access to deep lesions by way of well-designed long tips, and similarly improved tips may provide advantages in furcation areas. Some studies suggest less postoperative discomfort and less cementum removal with ultrasonics, but these findings are not universally demonstrated and devices in common use outside rigid study protocols are typically used suboptimally. Clearly, more research is needed in this area.

Although mechanical therapy, hand instrumentation or ultrasonic debridement, is the most common therapy for periodontitis of varying severity and has well-documented efficacy, there is a price to pay for this successful therapy, that is, the considerable amount of time and cost involved, the high level of operator skill needed, and some unavoidable discomfort for the patient. Based on these considerations, the short treatment regimes, which include full-mouth ultrasonic debridement that is completed within a few hours, may constitute a significant paradigm shift in periodontal practice.[44]

Initially, the objective of scaling and root planing was to remove soft and hard deposits, such as microbial biofilm and calculus, from the periodontal pocket and considerable amounts of infected cementum or even dentin from the root surface. The rationale behind this treatment was to eliminate bacterial endotoxins penetrating into the cementum[45,46] and thus establish local conditions ideal for soft-tissue healing. However, recent data point out that endotoxins do not penetrate into the cementum, but on the contrary, they loosely adhere to the surface of the root cementum.[47,48] Although, the necessity for removal of root substance is questioned,[49,50] a fairly smooth root surface does not retain microbial plaque and is thus a useful goal following instrumentation, but intentional and focused removal of root cementum is not necessary. On this basis, the use of instruments that disrupt the biofilm and remove deposits from a periodontal pocket, while causing minimal mechanical trauma to the structure of the root, is considered highly advantageous and ultrasonic devices are effective to this end.[51,52]

There are no categorical reports that newer designs of powered instruments are more advantageous than the conventional ultrasonic devices or that slimmer tip designs improve clinical outcomes compared with the traditional inserts.[53] Despite slimmer tip designs having better access to the narrow and deep periodontal pocket and minimizing soft tissue trauma during debridement, in vitro studies suggest that mechanical inefficiencies result from variations in the load applied to the tip and the flow rate of the irrigant. Walmsley and co-workers[43] (in 2008) reported that there is a need for manufacturers to use quality control programs and undertake clinical assessment studies before promoting these new technologies. Such studies would help instruct clinicians in their use and selection of power driven designs.

HOST RESPONSE CHANGES FOLLOWING PERIODONTAL THERAPY

Many studies have sought to determine the changes in antibody titers to putative periodontal pathogens following treatment. These changes can provide criteria on which to evaluate periodontal treatment and prognosis. Quirynen and colleagues[23] observed that 7 out of 11 patients, whose body temperature rose to more than 37°C after the second day of the one-stage full-mouth scaling and root planing, with or without the use of chlorhexidine treatment, had an overall pocket depth reduction exceeding 3.5 mm, whereas this was noted for only 4 of the remaining 13 patients that did not have an increase in temperature. Patients with an increase in body temperature on the evening after the second day of the full-mouth treatment had the more impressive clinical improvements, which was considered by the investigators to be due to an increased immunologic reaction. The investigators speculated that this might be the beneficial aspect of this treatment strategy.

One study investigated this hypothesis and frequent blood samples were taken from patients (biweekly intervals) over a longer period (overall 6 months) than had previously been done.[54] The data showed that although full-mouth instrumentation was completed in a shorter period (12 rather than 24 hours), no significant differences in the IgG antibody titers against 5 putative periodontal pathogens were detected compared with the standard quadrant root planing at biweekly intervals over a period of 6 months. Fortnightly sessions of quadrant root planing probably result in a similar host immune response to 12- or 24-hour full-mouth treatment, even though the latter treatment approach would be expected to have a greater potential for repeated inoculation of bacteria into the host tissues, thus eliciting a stronger immune response. Although IgG antibody titers were similar for both treatment groups, a significantly greater reduction in the antibody levels for *Prevotella intermedia* and *Treponema denticola* was seen between baseline and the initial reassessment (6 weeks after the completion of the instrumentation) for the full-mouth treated group compared with the quadrant group. When the changes in the serum antibody response over the course of treatment were considered within each treatment group, significant reductions in the IgG antibody levels for *P intermedia* and *T denticola* were seen between baseline and the initial reassessment for the full-mouth group, but this was not found for the quadrantwise group. These findings imply that same-day full-mouth treatment seems to have a stronger short-term effect on the systemic antibody response compared with the classical therapy of quadrant root planing at biweekly intervals, which complies with later data by Wang and colleagues.[55] However, the clinical significance of this finding is difficult to assess. The authors experience is that short-term perturbations of antibody responses occur during the active phase of periodontal therapy, but they show great variation across subjects and are therefore, difficult to meaningfully interpret.

CHANGES IN MICROBIAL PARAMETERS FOLLOWING THERAPY

The analysis of the microbiological parameters demonstrated that when identification methods based on molecular biology techniques were used to determine the quantity or the detection frequency of putative periodontal pathogens in subgingival plaque, no significant differences were found between the full-mouth approach and the quadrantwise treatment.[35,56,57] These data contrast with findings of De Soete and colleagues[58] who used DNA-DNA hybridization techniques and reported greater reductions in the "red" and "orange" complex bacteria for the full-mouth treatment modality. In a similar manner, additional studies that come from the University of Leuven using conventional culturing techniques[21,23,59,60] disagree with reports from researchers in Glasgow,[56] Tokyo[35] and Bonn,[57] which makes the interpretation of this inconsistency difficult.

In conclusion, it is difficult to compare the results obtained from various microbiological identification methods, which led Lang and co-workers[61] to decide not to meta-analyze microbiological results of the full-mouth treatment concept in a systematic review undertaken for the 6th European Workshop on Periodontology. The investigators pointed out that if recolonization of the already scaled sites was prevented by the full-mouth treatment, then the study of Jervøe-Storm and colleagues[57] that examined changes in the quantity of putative periodontal pathogens in subgingival plaque by elaborated laboratory methods should have validated this hypothesis, but did not do so.

In any therapy directed against microbes, the true commensals and pathogens involved in the disease process and the differential effects of treatment on these bacteria should be understood. A further complication exists in dealing with dental plaque, because this is the canonical example of a microbial biofilm in which it is estimated that up to 150 different microbial species may thrive, with many in a dormant form and thus resistant to antimicrobial therapies typically aimed at planktonic bacteria. The mechanical disruption of the microbial plaque biofilm offers considerable advantages over chemotherapeutic approaches. Eradication of the microbial plaque biofilm is central to the treatment of periodontal disease and this emphasizes the significance of the professionally performed mechanical removal of the biofilm coupled with home care measures to establish high oral hygiene standards, which serve to reduce or prevent future disease.

PERIODONTAL POCKETS AS MICROBIAL RESERVOIRS

The one-stage full-mouth scaling and root planing without chlorhexidine was shown to be equally efficacious as the one-stage full-mouth disinfection therapy, and it was shown to be more beneficial in clinical and microbiological responses than the classic treatment of consecutive sessions of scaling and root planning in patients with advanced periodontitis.[23] Although no conclusions can be reached on whether the enhanced clinical outcome of the full-mouth therapy is due to the full-mouth root planing itself, or the adjunctive use of chlorhexidine products, or the combination of both treatment approaches,[24] these findings indicate that the primary source of bacterial translocation is the periodontal pocket. The investigators suggested that these considerations should be taken into account when split-mouth clinical trials are designed. Another study from the same laboratory demonstrated that the composition of the microflora around teeth significantly influenced the formation of the subgingival flora around implants, and this was more pronounced when teeth and implants were in the same jaw.[62] These data highlight the role of periodontal pockets as bacterial reservoirs.

In the study of Apatzidou and Kinane,[25] full-mouth scaling and root planing was completed in 12 instead of 24 hours, as described by Quirynen and colleagues.[19] Although the interval between initiation and completion of treatment was lessened and therefore the chances for bacterial recolonization were also reduced, no significant microbiological or clinical differences were found between the 2 treatment groups 6 months postscaling, to support the hypothesis of Quirynen and colleagues.[19] However, the participants in this study were highly motivated patients and maintained a high standard of plaque control. Several studies showed that meticulous plaque control can affect the clinical and microbiological parameters in moderate[63,64] and deep pockets.[65–67] These data emphasize the magnitude of oral hygiene measures on the subgingival environment. Haffajee and colleagues[68] suggested that the beneficial effects of supragingival plaque control on the composition of the supra- and subgingival microflora decreased the risk of disease initiation or recurrence in maintenance of patients with periodontitis.

In a review, Greenstein[69] comments on the theory that "bacterial translocation" from one site to another is prevented by full-mouth root planing in 24 hours, and he concludes that the "seeding effect" of subgingival pathogens is unclear based on findings in the literature and requires further clarification. It seems that the transfer of pathogens to another ecological habitat does not necessarily result in their successful colonization, because either the host response or the antagonistic bacteria minimizes the chances of bacterial survival. Also, colonization of an implant site may be made possible, because the implant is a newly formed surface in the oral cavity and it does not have an established bacterial flora compared with a treated tooth site with an altered microflora.

SUMMARY

The aims of the studies involved in the full-mouth treatment concept are of interest; Quirynen and co-workers took a microbiological viewpoint and examined whether full-mouth treatment would prevent recolonization of the already instrumented periodontal pockets. Apatzidou and co-workers approached this clinical question with an immunologic bias and initially set out to consider whether the full-mouth treatment strategy would augment the host response and hence offer a superior clinical outcome; however, their results failed to support this initial hypothesis and, indeed, the clinical premise of superiority over quadrant scaling. Wennstrom and colleagues reviewed the full-mouth concept from a cost-effectiveness standpoint, demonstrating that the 1-hour treatment protocol is more cost-effective. Summarizing these factors, although there is a potential for translocation of periodontal pathogens from one pocket to another, carefully performed plaque control measures, removal of the biofilm, changes in the subgingival environment, and host response induced by treatment, may all serve to prevent reinfection of the instrumented sites and thus relapse of periodontal disease.

There is a lack of convincing and consistent evidence in the literature that the full-mouth disinfection approach is superior to full-mouth scaling and root planing or the traditional quadrantwise therapy based on clinical, microbiological, and immunologic parameters. Thus, one can conclude that all 3 treatment options are equally recommended for debridement in the cause-related phase of periodontal therapy in patients with chronic periodontitis.[61] The disruption and removal of the microbial biofilm and the initiation and establishment of meticulous plaque control are the key elements for success in nonsurgical periodontal treatment. The clinician should select the treatment modality based on practical considerations related to time constraints, clinical workload, and patient preference. The full-mouth treatment approach, adequately performed, may be beneficial in combination with systemic antibiotics, especially for the management of specific patient groups (with aggressive or progressing forms of periodontitis). Moreover, no significant differences were found between scaling and root planing with the use of only hand instruments versus ultrasonic debridement and between quadrantwise versus full-mouth approaches.

The comparison of the efficacy of surgical and nonsurgical procedures revealed that scaling and root planing alone or in combination with flap procedures are effective methods for the treatment of chronic periodontitis.[16] Also, the consistent message is that in treating deep pockets, open-flap debridement results in greater PPD reduction and clinical attachment gain than nonsurgical modalities. Nonsurgical modalities in shallower pockets consistently involve less post-therapy recession and are clearly recognized as being more conservative. Research is still needed on the clinical benefit of the granulation tissue removal that is a feature of periodontal surgical therapy and, to a lesser extent, occurs through indirect trauma in nonsurgical therapy.

REFERENCES

1. Badersten A, Nilvéus R, Egelberg J. Effect of nonsurgical periodontal therapy I. Moderately advanced periodontitis. J Clin Periodontol 1981;8:57–72.
2. Badersten A, Nilvéus R, Egelberg J. Effect of nonsurgical periodontal therapy II. Severely advanced periodontitis. J Clin Periodontol 1984;11:63–76.
3. Badersten A, Nilvéus R, Egelberg J. Effect of nonsurgical periodontal therapy III. Single versus repeated instrumentation. J Clin Periodontol 1984;11:114–24.
4. Badersten A, Nilveus R, Egelberg J. Effect of nonsurgical therapy (VIII). Probing attachment changes related to clinical characteristics. J Periodontol 1987;14: 425–32.
5. Knowles JW, Burgett FG, Nissle RR, et al. Results of periodontal treatment related to pocket depth and attachment level. Eight years. J Periodontol 1979;50:225–33.
6. Pihlstrom B, McHugh RB, Oliphant TH, et al. Comparison of surgical and nonsurgical treatment of periodontal disease. A review of current studies and additional results after 6 1/2 years. J Clin Periodontol 1983;10:524–41.
7. Ramfjord SP, Caffesse RG, Morrison EC, et al. 4 Modalities of periodontal treatment compared over 5 years. J Clin Periodontol 1987;14:445–52.
8. Cobb CM. Non-surgical pocket therapy: mechanical. Ann Periodontol 1996;1: 443–90.
9. Hill RW, Ramfjord SP, Morisson EC, et al. Four types of periodontal treatment compared over two years. J Periodontol 1981;52:655–62.

10. Lindhe J, Westfelt E, Nyman S, et al. Long-term effect of surgical/non-surgical treatment of periodontal disease. J Clin Periodontol 1984;11:448–58.
11. Lindhe J, Nyman S. Clinical trials in periodontal therapy. J Periodont Res 1987;22: 217–21.
12. Isidor F, Karring T, Attsröm R. The effect of root planing as compared to that of surgical treatment. J Clin Periodontol 1984;11:669–81.
13. Becker W, Becker BE, Caffesse R, et al. A longitudinal study comparing scaling, osseous surgery, and modified Widman procedures: results after 5 years. J Periodontol 2001;72:1675–84.
14. Antczak–Bouckoms A, Joshipura K, Burdick E, et al. Meta-analysis of surgical versus non-surgical methods of treatment for periodontal disease. J Clin Periodontol 1993;20:259–68.
15. Berkley CS, Antczak–Bouckoms A, Hoaglin DC, et al. Multiple–outcomes meta-analysis of treatments for periodontal disease. J Clin Periodontol 1995;74: 1031–9.
16. Heitz-Mayfield LJ, Trombelli L, Heitz F, et al. A systematic review of the effect of surgical debridement vs non-surgical debridement for the treatment of chronic periodontitis. J Clin Periodontol 2002;29(Suppl 3):92–102 [discussion: 160–2].
17. Lindhe J, Westfelt E, Nyman S, et al. Healing following surgical/non-surgical treatment of periodontal disease. A clinical study. J Clin Periodontol 1982;9:115–28.
18. Waerhaug J. Healing of the dento-epithelial junction following subgingival plaque control I. As observed in human biopsy material. J Periodontol 1978;49:1–8.
19. Quirynen M, Bollen CML, Vandekerckhove BNA, et al. Full- vs. partial-mouth disinfection in the treatment of periodontal infections: short-term clinical and microbiological observations. J Dent Res 1995;74:1459–67.
20. Vandekerckhove BN, Bollen CML, Dekeyser C, et al. Full- versus partial-mouth disinfection in the treatment of periodontal infections. Long-term clinical observations of a pilot study. J Periodontol 1996;67:1251–9.
21. Bollen CML, Mongardini C, Papaioannou W, et al. The effect of a one-stage full-mouth disinfection on different intra-oral niches. Clinical and microbiological observations. J Clin Periodontol 1998;25:56–66.
22. Mongardini C, van Steenberghe D, Dekeyser C, et al. One stage full- versus partial-mouth disinfection in the treatment of chronic adult or generalized early-onset periodontitis. I. Long-term clinical observations. J Periodontol 1999;70: 632–45.
23. Quirynen M, Mongardini C, De Soete M, et al. The rôle of chlorhexidine in the one-stage full-mouth disinfection treatment of patients with advanced adult periodontitis. J Clin Periodontol 2000;27:578–89.
24. Quirynen M, De Soete M, Boschmans G, et al. Benefit of "one-stage full-mouth disinfection" is explained by disinfection and root planing within 24 hours: a randomized controlled trial. J Clin Periodontol 2006;33:639–47.
25. Apatzidou DA, Kinane DF. Quadrant root planing versus same-day full-mouth root planing. I. Clinical findings. J Clin Periodontol 2004;31:132–40.
26. Jervøe-Storm P-M, Semaan E, AlAhdab H, et al. Clinical outcomes of quadrant root planing versus full-mouth root planing. J Clin Periodontol 2006;33:209–15.
27. Braatz L, Garrett S, Claffey N, et al. Antimicrobial irrigation of deep pockets to supplement non-surgical periodontal therapy. II. Daily irrigation. J Clin Periodontol 1985;12:630–8.
28. MacAlpine R, Magnusson I, Kiger R, et al. Antimicrobial irrigation of deep pockets to supplement oral hygiene instruction and root debridement. I. Bi-weeekly irrigation. J Clin Periodontol 1985;12:568–77.

29. Wennström JL, Heijl L, Dahlén G, et al. Periodic subgingival antimicrobial irrigation of periodontal pockets I. Clinical observations. J Clin Periodontol 1987;14: 541–50.
30. Wennström JL, Dahlén G, Gröndahl K, et al. Periodic subgingival antimicrobial irrigation of periodontal pockets II. Microbiological and radiographical observations. J Clin Periodontol 1987;14:573–80.
31. Lander PE, Newcomb GM, Seymour GJ, et al. The antimicrobial and clinical effects of a single subgingival irrigation of chlorhexidine in advanced periodontal lesions. J Clin Periodontol 1986;13:74–80.
32. Oosterwaal PJM, Mikx FHM, van 't Hof MA, et al. Short-term bactericidal activity of chlorhexidine gel, stannous fluoride gel and amine fluoride gel tested in periodontal pockets. J Clin Periodontol 1991;18:97–100.
33. Apatzidou DA. One stage full-mouth disinfection – treatment of choice? Letter to the editor. J Clin Periodontol 2006;33:942–3.
34. Quirynen M, Teughels W, van Steenberghe D. Impact of antiseptics on one-stage, full-mouth disinfection. Letter to the editor. J Clin Periodontol 2006;33:49–52.
35. Koshy G, Kawashima Y, Kiji M, et al. Effects of single-visit full-mouth ultrasonic debridement versus quadrant-wise ultrasonic debridement. J Clin Periodontol 2005;32:734–43.
36. Wennström JL, Tomasi C, Bertelle A, et al. Full-mouth ultrasonic debridement versus quadrant scaling and root planing as an initial approach in the treatment of chronic periodontitis. J Clin Periodontol 2005;32:851–9.
37. Copulos TA, Low SB, Walker CB, et al. Comparative analysis between a modified ultrasonic tip and hand instruments on clinical parameters of periodontal disease. J Periodontol 1993;64:694–700.
38. Kocher T, König J, Hansen P, et al. Subgingival polishing compared to scaling with steel curettes: a clinical pilot study. J Clin Periodontol 2001;28:194–9.
39. Kerry GJ. Roughness of root surfaces after use of ultrasonic instruments and hand curettes. J Periodontol 1967;38:340–6.
40. Dragoo MR. A clinical evaluation of hand and ultrasonic instruments on subgingival debridement. 1. With unmodified and modified ultrasonic inserts. Int J Periodontics Restorative Dent 1992;12:310–23.
41. Drisko CH. Trends in surgical and nonsurgical periodontal treatment. J Am Dent Assoc 2000;131:31S–8S.
42. Tunkel J, Heinecke A, Flemmig TF. A systematic review of efficacy of machine-driven and manual subgingival debridement in the treatment of chronic periodontitis. J Clin Periodontol 2002;29(Suppl 3):72–81 [discussion: 90–1].
43. Walmsley AD, Lea SC, Landini G, et al. Advances in power driven pocket/root instrumentation. J Clin Periodontol 2008;35(Suppl 8):22–8.
44. Kinane DF. Single-visit, full-mouth ultrasonic debridement: a paradigm shift in periodontal therapy? J Clin Periodontol 2005;32:732–3.
45. Hartfield CG, Baumhammers A. Cytotoxic effects of periodontally involved surfaces of human teeth. Arch Oral Biol 1971;16:465–8.
46. Aleo JJ, De Renzis FA, Farber PA, et al. The presence and biologic activity of cementum-bound endotoxin. J Periodontol 1974;45:672–5.
47. Hughes FJ, Auger DW, Smales FC. Investigation of the distribution of cementum-associated lipopolysaccharides in periodontal disease by scanning electron microscope immunohistochemistry. J Periodont Res 1988;23:100–6.
48. Cadosch J, Zimmermann U, Ruppert M, et al. Root surface debridement and endotoxin removal. J Periodont Res 2003;38:229–36.

49. Nyman S, Sarhed G, Ericsson I, et al. Role of "diseased" root cementum in healing following treatment of periodontal disease. An experimental study in the dog. J Periodont Res 1986;21:496–503.
50. Nyman S, Westfelt E, Sarhed G, et al. Role of "diseased" root cementum in healing following treatment of periodontal disease. A clinical study. J Clin Periodontol 1988;15:464–8.
51. Busslinger A, Lampe K, Beuchat M, et al. A comparative in vitro study of a magnetostrictive and a piezoelectric ultrasonic scaling instrument. J Clin Periodontol 2001;28:642–9.
52. Schmidlin PR, Beuchat M, Busslinger A, et al. Tooth substance loss resulting from mechanical, sonic and ultrasonic root instrumentation assessed by liquid scintillation. J Clin Periodontol 2001;28:1058–66.
53. Sanz M, Teughels W. Innovations in non-surgical periodontal therapy: consensus report of the Sixth European Workshop on Periodontology. J Clin Periodontol 2008;35(Suppl 8):3–7.
54. Apatzidou DA, Kinane DF. Quadrant root planing versus same-day full-mouth root planing. III. Dynamics of the immune response. J Clin Periodontol 2004;31:152–9.
55. Wang D, Koshy G, Nagasawa T, et al. Antibody response after single-visit full-mouth ultrasonic debridement versus quadrant-wise therapy. J Clin Periodontol 2006;33:632–8.
56. Apatzidou DA, Riggio MP, Kinane DF. Quadrant root planing versus one-day full-mouth root planing II. Microbiological findings. J Clin Periodontol 2004;31:141–8.
57. Jervøe-Storm P-M, AlAhdab H, Semaan E, et al. Microbiological outcomes of quadrant root planning *versus* full-mouth root planning as monitored by real-time PCR. J Clin Periodontol 2007;34:156–63.
58. De Soete M, Mongardini C, Pauwels M, et al. One-stage full-mouth disinfection. Long-term microbiological results analyzed by checkerboard DNA-DNA hybridization. J Periodontol 2001;72:374–82.
59. Bollen CML, Vandekerckhove BNA, Papaioannou W, et al. Full- versus partial-mouth disinfection in the treatment of periodontal infections. A pilot study: long-term microbiological observations. J Clin Periodontol 1996;23:960–70.
60. Quirynen M, Mongardini C, Pauwels M, et al. One stage full- versus partial-mouth disinfection in the treatment of chronic adult or generalized early-onset periodontitis. II. Long-term impact on microbial load. J Periodontol 1999;70:646–56.
61. Lang NP, Tan WC, Krähenmann MA, et al. A systematic review of the effects of full-mouth debridement with and without antiseptics in patients with chronic periodontitis. J Clin Periodontol 2008;35(Suppl 8):8–21.
62. Quirynen M, Papaioannou W, van Steenberghe D. Intraoral transmission and colonisation of oral hard surfaces. J Periodontol 1996;67:986–93.
63. McNabb H, Mombelli A, Lang NP. Supragingival cleaning 3 times a week. The microbiological effects in moderately deep pockets. J Clin Periodontol 1992;19:348–56.
64. Ximénez-Fyvie LA, Haffajee AD, Som S, et al. The effect of repeated professional supragingival plaque removal on the composition of the supra- and subgingival microbiota. J Clin Periodontol 2000;27:637–47.
65. Smulow JB, Turesky SS, Hill RG. The effect of supragingival plaque removal on anaerobic bacteria in deep periodontal pockets. J Am Dent Assoc 1983;107:737–42.
66. Dahlén G, Lindhe J, Sato K, et al. The effect of supragingival plaque control on the subgingival microbiota in subjects with periodontal disease. J Clin Periodontol 1992;19:802–9.

67. Hellström M-K, Ramberg P, Krok L, et al. The effect of supragingival plaque control on the subgingival microflora in human periodontitis. J Clin Periodontol 1996;23:934–40.
68. Haffajee AD, Smith C, Torresyap G, et al. Efficacy of manual and powered toothbrushes (II). Effect on microbiological parameters. J Clin Periodontol 2001;28:947–54.
69. Greenstein G. Full-mouth therapy versus individual quadrant root planning: a critical commentary. J Periodontol 2002;73:797–812.

Non-Surgical Chemotherapeutic Treatment Strategies for the Management of Periodontal Diseases

Joe W. Krayer, DDS, MS[a], Renata S. Leite, DMD, MS[a,c],
Keith L. Kirkwood, DDS, PhD[b,c,*]

KEYWORDS

- Periodontics • Antibiotics • Antiseptics
- Host-modulatory agent

Periodontal disease is a chronic infection of the periodontium affecting soft and mineralized tissues surrounding the teeth. Periodontal disease progression is associated with subgingival bacterial colonization and biofilm formation that provokes chronic inflammation of soft tissues, degradation of collagen fibers supporting the tooth to the gingiva and alveolar bone, and resorption of the alveolar bone itself. The fundamental role of microorganisms as the cause of periodontal disease was systematically demonstrated some 40 years ago, and research efforts have long focused on identifying the pathogenic microorganisms and their virulence factors.[1] The search for these putative microorganisms was driven, in part, by knowledge indicating that colonization of the oral cavity by commensal bacteria and the presence of dental biofilm is normally associated with health, similar to the colonization of the colon. In contrast, the microflora associated with periodontal disease was found to differ, with the biofilm dominated by anaerobic bacteria and spirochetes. To treat periodontal diseases as an infectious disease, numerous therapeutic strategies aimed at eradication of

This work was supported by P20RR017696 and R01DE018290 from the National Institutes of Health.

[a] Department of Stomatology, College of Dental Medicine, Medical University of South Carolina, 30 Bee Steet – room 115, Charleston, SC 29425, USA

[b] Department of Craniofacial Biology, College of Dental Medicine, Medical University of South Carolina, 173 Ashley Avenue, BSB 449, Charleston, SC 29425, USA

[c] Center for Oral Health Research, Medical University of South Carolina, 30 Bee Steet – room 115, Charleston, SC 29425, USA

* Corresponding author. Department of Craniofacial Biology, College of Dental Medicine, Medical University of South Carolina, 173 Ashley Avenue, BSB 449, Charleston, SC 29425.
E-mail address: klkirk@musc.edu (K.L. Kirkwood).

periodontal pathogens have been studied for many years, including local and systemic delivery of antimicrobial and antibiotic agents. This review provides an update on the chemotherapeutic agents used adjunctively to treat and manage periodontal diseases.

In the current paradigm of periodontal disease, specific periodontal pathogens are necessary for disease initiation; however, the extent and severity of tissue destruction are largely dependent on the nature of the host-microbial interactions. These interactions are dynamic, because both the microbial composition of the dental biofilm and the competency of host immune responses can vary, in the same individual, with time. This concept was developed in parallel to the advances on the understanding of the immune response, and research on periodontal disease has focused on the mechanisms of host-microbial interactions to understand the disease process and for the development of novel therapeutic strategies. For the past 2 decades, the host response to the bacterial challenge originating from the dental biofilm has been considered to play a major role on initiation of the disease and on the tissue destruction associated with its progress.[2] The importance of host-microbial interactions is reinforced by epidemiologic data indicating different susceptibilities to periodontal disease among individuals, despite the long-term presence of oral biofilm.[3–5] Other studies showing increased susceptibility and greater severity of periodontal disease in individuals with impaired immune response caused by systemic conditions also indicate the significance of the host response to the bacterial challenge.[6,7] Past and future directions of host-modulatory agents are addressed here to provide the dental practitioner with a broader prospective on the use of chemotherapeutic agents used to manage periodontal diseases.

SYSTEMIC ANTIBIOTICS

Traditional periodontal therapies have focused on the mechanical debridement of the root surfaces to maintain a healthy sulcus or produce an environment suitable for new attachment. The inability of mechanical treatment to always produce a desirable root surface coupled with the nature and complexity of the subgingival biofilm has fueled the search for adjunctive treatment regimens that increase the likelihood of successfully management of periodontal diseases.

Although more than 700 bacterial species may be present in the gingival sulcus, it is clear that only a subset of bacterial species are consistently found to be associated with diseased sites. These findings make the prospect of targeted antibiotic therapy an attractive goal. A thorough review of the microbiology of periodontal diseases is beyond the scope of this article; the reader is referred to the many reviews on this topic.[8]

Systemic antibiotic therapy has the obvious advantage of generally conventional and acceptable delivery, especially if oral administration is used. Shortcomings to oral administration include issues of patient adherence to dosing recommendations and the variable absorption of the antibiotic from the gastrointestinal tract. Moreover, it is difficult to be certain that the antibiotic chosen will be effective against the periodontal pathogens present in the sulcus unless culture and sensitivity tests have been completed. Culture and sensitivity tests are particularly useful for those cases that do not respond well to conventional mechanical therapy and/or commonly chosen antibiotic regimens. Another factor that is often overlooked is that systemic antibiotics do not penetrate the subgingival biofilm to kill bacteria. **Table 1** provides an overview of some orally active systemic antibiotics commonly used in clinical periodontics.

Table 1
Systemic antibiotics often used as adjuncts to mechanical periodontal therapy

Antibiotic Class	Agent	Effect	Target Organisms	Limitation
Penicillin	Amoxicillin	Bacteriocidal	Gram + and gram −	Penicillinase sensitive Patient hypersensitivity
	Augmentin	Bacteriocidal	Narrower spectrum than amoxicillin	More expensive than amoxicillin
Tetracycline	Tetracycline Minocycline Doxycycline	Bacteriostatic Bacteriostatic Bacteriostatic	Gram + > gram − Gram + > gram − Gram + > gram −	Bacterial resistance
Quinolone	Ciprofloxacin	Bacteriocidal	Gram − rods	Nausea, gastrointestinal discomfort
Macrolide	Azithromycin	Bacteriostatic OR bacteriocidal depending on concentration	Broad spectrum	
Lincomycin	Clindamycin	Bacteriocidal	Anaerobic bacteria	
Nitroimidazole	Metronidazole	Bacteriocidal to gram −	Gram −; especially *Porphyromonas gingivalis* and *Prevotella intermedia*	Not good choice for *A actinomycetemcomitans* infections

Based on the known spectrum of action of an antibiotic and the cumulative research profiling the bacterial species in the sulcus, it is possible to choose an antibiotic that should be an effective pharmacologic agent. However, caution should be used because none of these antibiotics is effective as a monotherapy to treat periodontal diseases. A systemically administered antibiotic will not produce the same effective concentration in the gingival sulcus as it might at another infected body site. Systemic antibiotics reach the periodontal tissues by transudation across serum, then cross the crevicular and junctional epithelia to enter the gingival sulcus. The concentration of the antibiotic in this site may be inadequate for the desired antimicrobial effect without mechanical disruption of the plaque biofilm. In addition to any effect produced in the sulcus, a systemically administered antibiotic will produce antimicrobial effects in other areas of the oral cavity. This additional effect will reduce bacterial counts on the tongue and other mucosal surfaces, thus potentially delaying in re-colonization of subgingival sites by the offending bacteria. However, research indicates that antibiotics are detectable in the gingival sulcus and the range of their concentrations in the gingival cervicular fluid is known to be in the therapeutic range for treatment efficacy. **Table 2** provides information to facilitate the clinician's decision to the most reasonable choice of antibiotic, dose, and duration of administration.

Many studies have described the effect of systemic antibiotic therapy on periodontal disease. Several different treatment regimens have been used successfully to manage periodontal diseases. It is not the intent of this discussion to review all the published studies in this area. The interested reader is referred to one of the many excellent, exhaustive reviews.[10] From many studies, it can be stated generally that systemic antibiotic therapy has little effect on supragingival plaque accumulation with a possible exception in one study where doxycycline significantly decreased plaque accumulation at a 12-week evaluation compared with placebo.[11]

Except for the combination of metronidazole with amoxicillin, systemic antibiotic treatment produces no clinically significant effects on periodontal pocket depth reduction compared with controls. The combination of metronidazole and amoxicillin has been found to produce more pocket depth reduction than control medication.[12] A 7-day regimen of systemic metronidazole significantly reduced the percentage of sites with bleeding compared with controls.[13] Others have reported a 12-month reduction in bleeding after treatment with a metronidazole-amoxicillin combination compared with a placebo treatment.[14] With respect to clinical attachment levels, systemic

Table 2
Systemic antibiotic dosing regimens

Antibiotic Agent	Regimen	Dosage and Duration
Single agent		
Amoxicillin	500 mg	Three times per day for 8 d
Azithromycin	500 mg	Once daily for 4–7 d
Ciprofloxacin	500 mg	Twice daily for 8 d
Clindamycin	300 mg	Three times daily for 10 d
Doxycycline or minocycline	100–200 mg	Once daily for 21 d
Metronidazole	500 mg	Three times daily for 8 d
Combination therapy		
Metronidazole + amoxicillin	250 mg of each	Three times daily for 8 d
Metronidazole + ciprofloxacin	500 mg of each	Twice daily for 8 d

metronidazole and combinations of metronidazole with other antibiotics have shown improvement in several studies. Several investigators found significant improvement of attachment levels at sites initially 4 to 6 mm in depth with a 7-day treatment with metronidazole.[15–17] Winkel and colleagues[12] showed that the combination of metronidazole and amoxicillin for 7 to 14 days produced a significant increase in the percentage of sites showing improved attachment levels compared with control sites. A combination of metronidazole and clindamycin for 3 weeks also produced improved attachment levels.[18,19]

Some data to date support a clinical benefit from the use of azithromycin as a systemic approach in combination with mechanical routines. In 1 limited study, 17 subjects receiving azithromycin (500 mg), 3 days before full-mouth scaling and root planing (SRP) produced greater clinical improvement than in 17 subjects treated with full-mouth SRP only.[19] Dastoor and colleagues[20] studied 30 patients who reported smoking more than 1 pack per day and presented with periodontitis. A comparison was made between the response to treatment with periodontal surgery and 500 mg azithromycin per day for 3 days and treatment with periodontal surgery only. The addition of azithromycin did not enhance improvement seen in both groups for attachment gain, depth reduction, and reduction of bleeding on probing. However, the adjunctive use of azithromycin was associated with a lower gingival index at 2 weeks and what the investigators saw as more rapid wound healing. The addition of azithromycin also produced reductions of red-complex bacteria that were maintained for up to 3 months.

The combination of amoxicillin (375 mg)/metronidazole (500 mg), each taken 3 times per day for 7 days in conjunction with full-mouth periodontal debridement performed within a 48-hour period, produced more favorable clinical effects than the same full-mouth debridement routine alone. In the subjects treated with the antibiotics, probing depths showed a greater reduction with fewer bleeding sites on probing and a smaller number of sites requiring additional therapy at 6 months following initial therapy.[21]

A reasonable choice of a systemic antibiotic routine, particularly in the absence of culture and sensitivity testing, may be the combination metronidazole and amoxicillin, 250 to 500 mg of each, taken 3 times per day for 8 days. Another reasonable choice may be the combination of metronidazole and ciprofloxacin, 500 mg of each, taken twice daily for 8 days. This combination adds the benefit of treatment of infections with *Aggregatibacter actinomycetemcomitans*.

Concerns are frequently raised regarding bacterial resistance with systemic antibiotic therapy.[22] This has the potential to eliminate a possibly important or critical drug from the possible treatment options for diseases with more life-threatening potential than the risk of ongoing periodontal disease. It is important to remember that systemic antibiotic therapy is not intended as a monotherapy but is always best as an adjunctive therapy combined with mechanical therapy and plaque control. Management of severe types of periodontitis should not rely only on systemic antibiotics used in conjunction with mechanical debridement but may require the subgingival administration of antiseptics and/or local antibiotics and periodontal surgery.[10]

LOCAL ANTIBIOTIC THERAPY

After considering the risk to benefit ratio of systemic antibiotic administration as a treatment of periodontal diseases, interest in local delivery of antibiotics developed (**Table 3**). Historically, the first such local antibiotic therapy for periodontal disease was the Actisite (no longer commercially available) fiber system. Actisite was supplied as hollow, nonabsorbable fibers filled with tetracycline (12.7 mg in

Table 3
Local antibiotic delivery systems

Antimicrobial Agent	Delivery Form	Drawback	GCF Concentration	Time to Absorption	Brand Name
Tetracycline 12.7 mg per 23 cm (9 in) of fiber	Hollow fibers	Must be removed	>1300 μg/mL for 10 d	Not absorbable	Actisite, not commercially available
10% Doxycycline	Fluid; multisite depending on volume of site; in syringe	Often pulls out when removing syringe	250 μg/mL still noted at 7 d	21 d	Atridox
25% Metronidazole gel	Fluid; multisite depending on volume of site; in syringe	May require multiple applications for desirable results	More than 120 mg/mL of sulcus fluid in the first few hours	Concentration decreases rapidly after the first few hours[9]	Elyzol
2% Minocycline spheres	Solid; in unit doses applied with syringe	Unit doses may not be sufficient for every site volume	Therapeutic drug levels for 14 d	14 d	Arestin
0.5% Azithromycin	Gel in syringe		Peak at 2 h at 2041 μg/mL decreased from 324 μg/mL on day 7 to 3 μg/mL on day 28	Still present at 28 d	Not commercially available

23 cm (9 in) fiber). The fiber was inserted into the pocket, wrapped repeatedly circumferentially around the tooth keeping the fiber in the pocket. Often a periodontal dressing was placed to help keep the fiber in the pocket. The fiber was retained for 10 days until removed by the operator. During this 10-day period drug concentrations of more than 1300 µg/ml of tetracycline were achieved and maintained. When the fiber was removed the soft tissue was often distended allowing temporary improved access and visibility of the root surfaces for any additional root planing or calculus removal. Following removal of the fiber the soft tissues generally showed shrinkage, reduction of depth, and a reduction of the clinical signs of inflammation. The Actisite system, although very effective, was tedious to use and required a second visit for removal of the fiber. These issues fueled the development of absorbable systems for antibiotic delivery.

The first resorbable local antibiotic system was Atridox (Atrix Laboratories, Fort Collins, CO). In this system, longer half-life doxycycline replaced tetracycline supplied at a concentration of 42.5 mg per unit dose of material. This system requires mixing powder and liquid components using 2 linked luer lock syringes. After adequate mixing, a blunt cannula is attached to 1 of the syringes and the material expressed from the syringe into the pocket. Atridox is absorbed after 7 days and reports of antibiotic concentrations of 250 µg/ml in the pocket have been reported. No second visit for removal of the material is necessary. The application of Atridox can be somewhat tedious as the material tends to pull out of the pocket when the syringe is removed. Retaining the material with a periodontal dressing can be helpful but is often unnecessary. Atridox improved the local antibiotic delivery by allowing placement of the material to the depth of most pockets and in a manner that allowed it to conform to the shape of the pocket unlike the solid fibers of Actisite. Depending on the size of the pocket, more than 1 site could be treated with a single unit dose of Atridox.

Further development of absorbable local antibiotic systems led to Arestin (OraPharma), which uses minocycline in a microsphere configuration, each sphere measuring 20 to 60 µm in diameter. Arestin is supplied in single-dose units that are applied into the pocket with a reusable, sterilizable syringe. Each unit dose contains 1 mg of mincocycline. The sphere is a bioabsorable polymer of poly(glycolide-co-DL-lactide), which is hydrolyzed into CO_2 and H_2O. The antibiotic maintains therapeutic drug levels and remains in the pocket for 14 days. This configuration of material allows placement to the depths of most pockets and although the material cannot conform to the shape of the pocket and the Atridox gel, it is still easier to use than the solid Actisite fibers.

Another material, not now available in the United States, is Elyzol (Colgate), a metronidazole gel system. Elyzol is supplied as 25% metronidazole in a glyceryl monooleate and sesame oil base. The concentration of metronidazole in this system is 250 mg/g of material that is applied as a gel using a syringe.

Overall efficacy of local antibiotic therapies has been evaluated using meta-analysis of 50 articles, each reporting studies of at least 6 months follow-up.[23] The meta-analysis considered studies of the addition of local adjuncts and found such additions provide generally favorable but minimal differences compared with SRP alone. Additional statistically significant depth reductions of 0.1 to 0.5 mm may be possible and smaller, less frequently statistically significant improvement in attachment levels were noted. The clinical effects of these various systems have been reported in several publications. **Table 4** summarizes several studies of various local adjunctive materials. The overall treatment effect is somewhat variable and, although found to be statistically significant, has not resulted in widespread use of these systems by the clinical community.

Table 4 Local antibiotic system studies				
Agent	Subjects	Depth Change with SRP only	Depth Change with SRP + Agent	Sites With at Least 2 mm Attachment Gain with SRP + Agent
Tetracycline fibers[24]	107	0.67	1.02 (fiber only)	Not reported
Doxycycline gel[25]	411	1.08	1.30 (drug only)	38% (drug only)
Doxycycline gel[26]	105	1.3	1.5	52%
Doxycycline gel[27]	48	1.5–2.19	1.63–2.29	34.4% vs 18.1% S/RP only
Minocycline spheres[28]	728	1.08	1.32	42%
Minocycline spheres[29]	127	1.01	1.38	Not reported; reports attachment gain of 1.16 with agent, 0.8 S/RP only
Metronidazole gel[30]	206	1.3	1.5 (drug only)	Not reported
Azithromycin gel[31]	80	2.13	2.53	Not reported; reports greater gain at all time points with agent

ANTISEPTICS

The use of chemical agents with antiplaque or antigingivitis action as adjuncts to oral hygiene seems to be of limited value, because mouth rinses do not penetrate appreciably into the gingival crevice, but they show specific benefits when used as adjuncts to control gingival inflammation, especially in acute situations, postsurgically, and during periods of interrupted hygiene.[32] The American Dental Association (ADA) seal of acceptance is seen as a standard for oral health care products. The ADA Seal Program ensures that professional and consumer dental products meet rigorous ADA criteria for safety and effectiveness. Guidelines have been established for the control of gingivitis and supragingival plaque (http://www.ada.org/ada/seal/index.asp). These guidelines describe the clinical, biologic, and laboratory studies necessary to evaluate safety and effectiveness and are subject to revision at any time (**Box 1**). The guidelines do not describe criteria for evaluating the management of periodontitis or other periodontal diseases. All claims of efficacy, including health benefit claims (eg, gingivitis reduction), and claims that imply a health benefit (eg, plaque reduction) must be documented. There will be two Seal statements to be used with an accepted product, depending on whether or not the product's mechanism of action is related to plaque reduction.

The challenge for chemical plaque control is to develop an active antiplaque agent that does not disturb the commensal microflora of the oral cavity. Oral antiseptics have evolved from short-lived (effective soon after rinsing) first-generation antimicrobials (**Table 5**), to second-generation products, which have antimicrobial effects that last for a longer time period after the mouth rinse has been expectorated (**Table 6**).

Box 1
Guidelines for ADA acceptance of chemotherapeutic products for the control of gingivitis and supragingival dental plaque (http://www.ada.org/ada/seal/index.asp)

Product efficacy must be demonstrated by 2 independent, well-designed, 6-month clinical studies using a placebo control and conducted by independent investigators.

All published studies assessing the effectiveness of the product must be referenced, including studies that do not show any effect.

All proprietary studies, including those that do not show any effect, must also be provided.

Studies should assess the ability of a chemotherapeutic agent to prevent or reduce gingivitis and to inhibit or reduce plaque formation or plaque pathogenicity.

Masked studies are required; uniquely labeled products must be used and group coding must be avoided.

At least 1 study shall be conducted on a US population.

Populations selected for the studies must be representative of individuals for whom the product is intended, which, in most cases, would be individuals with mild to moderate gingivitis.

Trials must report all treatment groups.

Statistically significant reductions in both the clinical manifestations of gingivitis and in the inhibition or reduction of plaque or plaque pathogenicity related to gingivitis must be demonstrated.

Reductions relative to plaque and gingivitis should be demonstrated after 6 months of use in 2 studies and be measured against a placebo control rather than baseline scores.

The product must show clinical significance in gingivitis reduction compared with placebo controls in at least 2 clinical studies.

Microbiological sampling should estimate plaque qualitatively to complement indices that measure plaque quantitatively.

Gingivitis measurements shall demonstrate:

1. that the estimated proportionate reductions (ie, [control−active]/control) be no less than 15% in favor of the active treatment with a confidence interval of $\pm 10\%$, and statistically significant in each of at least 2 studies;

2. that, in addition, the (arithmetical) mean of the estimated proportionate reductions (ie, [control−active]/control) across the above studies be no less than 20%.

Plaque measurements shall demonstrate that quantitative plaque reductions or reductions in plaque pathogenicity for those products whose antigingivitis action is through plaque reduction or modifications are statistically significant.

The most likely mechanism(s) of action of the product should be given, with supporting data.

On the downside, it is also recognized that oral hygiene products may have the potential for producing harm in the mouth, some of which are more serious and long-lasting than others. Harms range from production of a cosmetic nuisance, such as staining resulting from the use of cationic antiseptics like chlorhexidine and cetylpyridinium chloride, to more permanent damage to the dental hard tissues through possible erosive and abrasive effects of low-pH mouth rinses and tooth-pastes, respectively. Of serious concern is controversially the ability to produce carcinogenic changes to the oral mucosa through the use of alcoholic mouth rinses. Recently, the potential harm of oral hygiene products to oral and systemic health was fully reviewed with reference to present-day evidence.[33]

Table 5
First-generation antimicrobials

Antimicrobial	Commercial Name	ADA Seal of Acceptance	Active Ingredients	Alcohol Content	Mechanism of Action	Efficacy Published by the Manufacturer
Phenolic compounds	Listerine (Johnson & Johnson)	Yes	Essential oils: - Thymol (0.06%) - Eucalyptol (0.09%) - Methyl salicylate (0.06%) - Menthol (0.04%)	26.9%	Seems to be related to alteration of the bacterial cell wall	52% plaque reduction 36% gingivitis reduction (http://www.listerine.com/)
Sanguinarine	Viadent (Colgate)	No	0.03% Sanguinarine extract	5.5%	Alteration of bacterial cell surfaces so that aggregation and attachment is reduced	28% plaque reduction 24% gingivitis reduction (http://www.colgateprofessional.com/products/Viadent-Advanced-Care-Oral-Rinse/details)
Quaternary ammonium compounds	Cepacol and Scope (Procter & Gamble)	No	Cepacol: 0.05% CPC Scope: 0.045% CPC + 0.005% domiphen bromide	Cepacol: 14% Scope: 18.9%	Related to increased bacterial cell wall permeability which favors lysis, decreased cell metabolism and a decreased ability for bacteria to attach to tooth surfaces	15.8% plaque reduction (http://www.cepacol.com/products/mouthwash.asp) and (http://www.pg.com/product_card/prod_card_main_scope.shtml) 15.4% gingivitis reduction

Abbreviation: CPC, cetylpyridinium chloride.

Table 6
Second-generation antimicrobials

Antimicrobial	Cetylpyridinium Chloride	Chlorhexidine
Commercial name	Crest Pro-Health (Procter & Gamble)	Peridex (3M Espe) Periogard (Colgate)
ADA seal of acceptance	No	Yes
Active ingredients	0.07% CPC	0.12% Chlorhexidine gluconate (http://solutions.3m.com/wps/portal/3M/en_US/preventive-care/home/products/home-care-therapies/peridex/) and (http://www.colgateprofessional.com/products/Colgate-Periogard-Rinse-Rx-only/details)
Mechanism of action	Bactericidal agent interacts with the bacterial membrane. The cellular pressure disrupts the cell membrane and effectively kills the bacteria	Positively charged chlorhexidine molecule binds to negatively charged microbial cell wall, altering osmotic equilibrium, causing potassium and phosphorus leakage, precipitation of cytoplasmic contents, and consequent cell death
Efficacy published by the manufacturer	Similar to Listerine (http://www.dentalcare.com/soap/products/index.htm)	Reduction in certain aerobic and anaerobic bacteria from 54 to 97% after 6 mo use (http://solutions.3m.com/wps/portal/3M/en_US/preventive-care/home/products/home-care-therapies/peridex/) - 29% gingivitis reduction - 54% plaque reduction (http://www.colgateprofessional.com/products/Colgate-Periogard-Rinse-Rx-only/details)

Abbreviation: CPC, cetylpyridinium chloride.

Phenolic Compounds

Among the first-generation antimicrobials, the phenolic compounds, such as Listerine and its generic version, are the only ones that have the ADA Seal of Acceptance to prevent and reduce supragingival plaque accumulation and gingivitis. Short-term studies have shown plaque and gingivitis reduction averaging 35%,[34] and long-term studies have shown plaque reduction between 13.8% and 56.3% and gingivitis reduction between 14% and 35.9%.[35,36] Possible adverse effects reported in the literature include a burning sensation, bitter taste, and possible staining of teeth.

Chlorhexidine

Chlorhexidine gluconate (0.12%), such as Peridex and Periogard, is sold in the United States by prescription only. It was the first antimicrobial shown to inhibit plaque formation and the development of chronic gingivitis.[37] Chlorhexidine is more effective against *gram*-positive than *gram*-negative bacteria. It does have antiyeast properties. It has low toxicity, because it is poorly absorbed from the gastrointestinal tract and 90% is excreted in the feces. Chlorhexidine 0.12% is indicated for short-term (< 2 months) use, intermittent short-term (alternating on and off every 1 to 2 months), and long-term (> 3 months to indefinitely) use (**Table 7**) depending on clinical indications. Of all the products included here, chlorhexidine seems to be the most effective agent for reduction of plaque and gingivitis, with short-term reductions averaging 60%.[38] Long-term reductions in plaque averaged between 45% and 61% and in gingivitis, 27% to 67%.[32] Adverse effects reported include staining of teeth, mucositis and reversible epithelial desquamation, alteration of taste, and increased supragingival calculus.[38,39]

Table 7
Chlorhexidine 0.12% indications

Short-Term Indication (< 2 months)	Intermittent Short-Term Indications (Alternating on and off every 1 to 2 months)	Long-Term Indications (> 3 months to Indefinitely)
Gingivitis	Gingivitis	Patients with reduced resistance to bacterial plaque: AIDS, leukemia, kidney disease, bone marrow transplants, agranulocytosis, thrombocytopenia
Following periodontal and oral surgery	Periodontal maintenance	Physically handicapped patients: rheumatoid arthritis, scleroderma, disturbance of muscles and/or motor capacity and coordination
During initial periodontal therapy	Physically and/or mentally handicapped	Patients treated with: cytotoxic drugs, immunosuppressive drugs, radiation therapy
Treatment of candidiasis	Extensive prosthetic reconstruction	

Other Antimicrobial Mouth Rinses

Several other agents have been evaluated for their effect on bacterial plaque and gingivitis, but results are inferior to those of chlorhexidine and phenolic compounds (**Table 8**). Pires and colleagues[41] have concluded that a mouthwash containing a combination of Triclosan/Gantrez and sodium bicarbonate has an in vitro antimicrobial activity superior to that of a placebo, but still inferior to that of chlorhexidine. Triclosan acts as a broad-spectrum biocide, targeting multiple nonspecific targets and causing disruption of bacterial cells. Although bacterial isolates with reduced susceptibility to Triclosan were produced in laboratory experiments by repeated exposure to sublethal concentrations of the agent,[42] the studies on oral-care formulations, like toothpastes and mouth rinses, report no significant changes in the microbial flora or the antimicrobial susceptibility of the microflora.[43,44]

Oxygenating agents have also been evaluated. Although their antiinflammatory properties result in less bleeding on probing, a major sign of periodontal inflammation, the bacteria causing the disease are not necessarily reduced.[45] Safety questions such as tissue injury and cocarcinogenicity have been raised with the chronic use of hydrogen peroxide.[46]

Table 9 shows studies comparing different mouth rinses used for plaque and gingivitis reduction. Chlorhexidine is reported as the gold standard with superior effectiveness compared with other mouth rinses and when the possible adverse effects are taken into consideration (see **Table 7**). If chlorhexidine is effective 60% of the time, the phenolic compounds are next in effectiveness, reducing plaque formation and gingivitis by about 35%. Sanguinarine and the quaternary ammonium compounds are next with 18% and 15%, respectively. The oxygenating agents are the least effective, showing 0% reduction in either plaque formation or gingivitis.

ANTIINFLAMMATORY AGENTS FOR MANAGEMENT OF PERIODONTAL DISEASE

It is well established that periodontal disease is an infectious disease and that the host immune and inflammatory response to the microbial challenge mediates tissue destruction.[48] Considering that the primary cause of the disease is the bacteria in plaque and their products, mechanical and chemical approaches to reduce the presence of periodontal pathogens in the plaque have been largely used in the treatment of periodontal patients for many years.[49] Most recently, a better understanding of the participation of host immune inflammatory mediators in disease progression has increased the investigation of the use of modulating agents as an adjunctive therapy to the periodontal treatment. Inhibition or blockade of proteolytic enzymes, proinflammatory mediators, and osteoclast activity have been outcomes measured following use of these agents, which has led to encouraging results in preclinical and clinical studies.[50] More specifically, 3 types of host-modulatory agents have been investigated for the management of periodontitis including antiproteinases, antiinflammatory agents, and antiresorptive agents.

One important group of proteolytic enzymes present in the periodontal tissues is the matrix metalloproteinases (MMPs), which include collagenases, gelatinases, and metalloelastases. MMPs are produced by many periodontal tissues and are responsible for remodeling the extracellular matrix.[51] In 1985, tetracyclines were found to have anticollagenolytic activity and proposed as potential host modulating agents for periodontal treatment.[52] Initial studies showed that doxycycline was the most potent tetracycline in inhibition of collagenolytic activities.[53] This property of doxycycline provided the pharmacologic rationale for the use of a low or subantimicrobial dose

Table 8
Other antimicrobial mouthrinses

Antimicrobial	Commercial Name	ADA Seal of Acceptance	Active Ingredients	Mechanism of Action	Efficacy
Oxygenating agents	Peroxyl (Colgate)	No	Hydrogen peroxide	Antiinflammatory properties reduce BOP, a major sign of inflammation; bacterial load is not necessarily reduced; bubbling action cleans and alleviates discomfort to promote healing	Long-term studies do not support effectiveness Short-term studies offer contradictory findings
Chlorine dioxide	RetarDEX (Periproducts) Oxyfresh	No	1% Chlorine dioxide	Stable, free radical and an oxidant with algicidal, bactericidal, cysticidal, fungicidal, sporicidal, and viricidal properties	Minimal plaque reduction, but has shown decreases in volatile sulfur compounds and halitosis
Zinc choride	Breath Rx	No	- Zinc chloride - Phenolic oils (thymol and eucalyptus oil)	Zinc has an affinity to sulfur and odorizes sulfhydryl groups with zinc ions forming stable mercaptides with the substrate, the precursors, and/or the volatile sulfur compounds directly	BreathRx is a scientific bad breath treatment specially designed to help treat the causes of bad breath and the symptoms
Triclosan	Not available in the United States	N/A	Triclosan	A low toxicity, nonionic phenolic derivative with a wide spectrum of antimicrobial and antiinflammatory activities[40]	In vitro studies show antimicrobial activity superior to that of a placebo, but inferior to that of chlorhexidine[41]

Table 9
Comparison studies

Antiseptics Compared	Methodology	Results	References
Listerine Viadent Peridex Placebo	31 volunteers with healthy gingiva ceased all oral hygiene procedures but rinsing with the designated mouth rinse for 21 d	Peridex was superior in its ability to maintain optimal gingival health throughout the period of use	Siegrist et al[47]
Listerine Peridex Placebo	Double-blind, controlled clinical trial. After a baseline complete dental prophylaxis, 124 healthy adults used the mouth rinse as a supplement to regular oral hygiene for 6 mo	Both Listerine and Peridex significantly inhibited development of plaque by 36.1% and 50.3%, respectively, and the development of gingivitis by 35.9% and 30.5% respectively, compared with placebo	Overholser et al[39]
Chlorhexidine 0.12% Hydrogen peroxide 1% Placebo	32 subjects ceased oral hygiene procedures, but rinsed, twice a day, with the designated mouth rinse for 21 d	The chlorhexidine group showed 95% reduction in gingivitis incidence, 100% reduction in BOP, and 80% reduction in plaque scores compared with placebo	Gusberti et al[45]

of doxycycline (SDD) that was shown to be efficient in inhibiting mammalian collagenase activity without developing antibiotic resistance.[54]

Several clinical studies have been conducted assessing the benefits of the SDD as an adjunctive therapy to SRP in the treatment of periodontal disease. Reddy and colleagues[50] recently presented a meta-analysis of 6 selected clinical studies comparing (long-term) systemic SDD (doxycycline 20 mg twice a day) with placebo controls in periodontal patients. A statistically significant adjunctive benefit on clinical attachment levels (CAL) and probing depth was found when SDD was used in combination with SRP, in both 4 to 6 mm and 7 mm or greater pocket depth categories. Bleeding on probing (BOP) was not assessed in the meta-analysis but, in general, SDD did not improve this parameter when compared with placebo. No significant adverse effects were reported in any of the studies.

The nonsteroidal antiinflammatory drugs (NSAIDs) represent the next major pharmacologic class of agents that has been well studied as inhibitors of the host response in periodontal disease. These agents are well known for the ability to prevent prostanoid formation. In this process, arachidonic acid liberated from membrane phospholipids of cells after tissue damage or stimulus is metabolically transformed via cyclooxygenase or lipoxygenase pathways in compounds with potent biologic activities.[48] The cyclooxygenase enzymes are recognized to have 2 isoforms: cyclo-oxygenase 1 (COX-1) which is a constitutive enzyme present in most cells, and cyclo-oxygenase 2 (COX-2), which is inducible and is present in cells involved in inflammation.[55] The cyclooxygenase pathway produces prostaglandins, prostacyclin, and thromboxane, called prostanoids. Some prostanoids have proinflammatory prop-erties and have been associated with destructive process in inflammatory diseases. In periodontal diseases, prostaglandin E_2 (PGE_2) levels have been found to be correlated with inflammation and bone resorption.[48] Its levels in gingival tissues and in the gingival crevicular fluid (GCF) have been shown to be significantly elevated in patients with periodontal disease compared with healthy patients.[56,57]

Recently, selective NSAIDs capable of inhibiting COX-2 without affecting constitu-tive isoform COX-1, have been found to share the same bone-sparing effects[58–61] without inducing the adverse effects associated with COX-1 suppression, such as gastroduodenal problems and renal toxicity. Several clinical trials have been con-ducted to test the effect of NSAIDs on periodontal status. In a systematic review,[50] 10 clinical studies, in which therapeutic outcomes of NSAIDs were expressed as CAL or alveolar crestal height as measured by subtraction radiography, were selected. In these studies various different NSAIDs were systemically or locally administered, including flurbiprofen, meclofenamate, ibuprofen, ketorolac, naproxen, and aspirin. Although the heterogeneity of data did not permit a meta-analysis, limited quantitative analysis tended to show alveolar bone maintenance when NSAIDs were combined with mechanical therapy. None of these studies found significantly less attachment loss after NSAID adjunctive therapy compared with SRP alone.

Alveolar bone loss or destruction is the hallmark feature of periodontal disease. The use of bone-sparing drugs that inhibit alveolar bone resorption is another facet of host-modulation therapy. Bisphosphonates are a class of agents that binds to the hydox-yapatite in the bone matrix to prevent matrix dissolution by interfering with osteoclast function through various direct and indirect mechanisms.[62] The principal therapeutic application for bisphosphonates is in the prevention and treatment of osteoporosis, and in the treatment of Paget disease and metastatic bone disease.[63] In periodontics, their use was proposed initially for diagnostic and therapeutic use. As therapeutic agents, bisphosphonates were shown to reduce alveolar bone loss and increase mineral density but not to improve other clinical conditions in animal periodontitis models.[64,65] Five studies that assessed the effect of bisphosphonates as an adjunc-tive agent to SRP in human periodontal treatment were found to date.[66–70] Alendro-nate was the bisphosphonate used in 4 studies for a period of 6 months. One study used risedronate for 12 months.[70] All the studies presented significant clinical improvement compared with placebo, including probing depth reduction, clinical attachment gain, reduction in BOP, alveolar bone gain and increase in bone mineral density. These results encourage the use of bisphosphonates as an adjunctive agent to periodontal therapy. Additional longer-term studies need to be implemented to confirm the benefits of these drugs.

Recently, high-dose and long-term use of bisphosphonates has been reported to be associated with osteonecrosis of the jaw (ONJ).[71,72] Data from multiple sour-ces indicate that patients with prior dental problems may have a higher risk of ONJ. However, as more data are being reported, whether bisphosphonates are causative for ONJ still remains controversial. Because bisphosphonates are potent osteoclast inhibitors, their long-term use may suppress bone turnover and compromise healing of even physiologic micro-injuries within bone.[73] Despite the encouraging therapeutic results in the management of periodontal disease, further long-term studies are warranted to determine the relative risk/benefit ratio of bisphosphonate therapy.

FUTURE NON-SURGICAL APPROACHES

Various treatment strategies have been developed to target the host response for the management of periodontitis. MMP inhibitors such as low-dose formulations of doxycycline have been used in combination with SRP[74] or surgical therapy.[75] In addition, high-risk patient populations such as patients with diabetes or recurrent periodontal disease have benefited from systemic MMP administration.[76–78] Encouraging results have been obtained following soluble antagonists of tumor necrosis factor (TNF) and IL-1 delivered locally to periodontal tissues in nonhuman primates.[79,80] Other therapeutic strategies that are being explored are aimed at inhibiting signal transduction pathways involved in inflammation. Pharmacologic inhibitors of NF-kB and p38 mitogen activating protein (MAP) kinase pathways are actively being developed to manage inflammatory bone diseases.[81,82] p38 inhibitors have already shown promise in preclinical models of periodontal diseases.[2,83] Using this novel strategy, inflammatory mediators including proinflammatory cytokines (IL-1, TNF, IL-6), MMPs, and others would be inhibited at the level of cell signaling pathways required for activation of the transcription factor necessary for inflammatory gene expression or mRNA stability. These therapies may provide the next generation of adjuvant chemotherapeutics to manage chronic periodontitis.

REFERENCES

1. Socransky SS, Haffajee AD. Evidence of bacterial etiology: a historical perspective. Periodontol 2000 1994;5:7–25.
2. Kirkwood KL, Cirelli JA, Rogers JE, et al. Novel host response therapeutic approaches to treat periodontal diseases. Periodontol 2000 2007;43:294–315.
3. Baelum V, Fejerskov O. Tooth loss as related to dental caries and periodontal breakdown in adult Tanzanians. Community Dent Oral Epidemiol 1986;14(6):353–7.
4. Baelum V, Wen-Min L, Fejerskov O, et al. Tooth mortality and periodontal conditions in 60–80-year-old Chinese. Scand J Dent Res 1988;96(2):99–107.
5. Loe H, Anerud A, Boysen H, et al. Natural history of periodontal disease in man. Rapid, moderate and no loss of attachment in Sri Lankan laborers 14 to 46 years of age. J Clin Periodontol 1986;13(5):431–45.
6. Feller L, Lemmer J. Necrotizing periodontal diseases in HIV-seropositive subjects: pathogenic mechanisms. J Int Acad Periodontol 2008;10(1):10–5.
7. Mealey BL. Impact of advances in diabetes care on dental treatment of the diabetic patient. Compend Contin Educ Dent 1998;19(1):41–4, 6–8, 50 passim [quiz 60].
8. Socransky SS, Haffajee AD. Periodontal microbial ecology. Periodontol 2000 2005;38:135–87.
9. Knoll-Kohler E. Metronidazole dental gel as an alternative to scaling and root planing in the treatment of localized adult periodontitis. Is its efficacy proved? Eur J Oral Sci 1999;107(6):415–21.
10. Slots J, Ting M. Systemic antibiotics in the treatment of periodontal disease. Periodontol 2000 2002;28:106–76.
11. Ng VW, Bissada NF. Clinical evaluation of systemic doxycycline and ibuprofen administration as an adjunctive treatment for adult periodontitis. J Periodontol 1998;69(7):772–6.

12. Winkel EG, Van Winkelhoff AJ, Timmerman MF, et al. Amoxicillin plus metronidazole in the treatment of adult periodontitis patients. A double-blind placebo-controlled study. J Clin Periodontol 2001;28(4):296–305.
13. Watts T, Palmer R, Floyd P. Metronidazole: a double-blind trial in untreated human periodontal disease. J Clin Periodontol 1986;13(10):939–43.
14. Lopez NJ, Gamonal JA, Martinez B. Repeated metronidazole and amoxicillin treatment of periodontitis. A follow-up study. J Periodontol 2000;71(1):79–89.
15. Loesche WJ, Giordano JR, Hujoel P, et al. Metronidazole in periodontitis: reduced need for surgery. J Clin Periodontol 1992;19(2):103–12.
16. Loesche WJ, Syed SA, Morrison EC, et al. Metronidazole in periodontitis. I. Clinical and bacteriological results after 15 to 30 weeks. J Periodontol 1984;55(6): 325–35.
17. Elter JR, Lawrence HP, Offenbacher S, et al. Meta-analysis of the effect of systemic metronidazole as an adjunct to scaling and root planing for adult periodontitis. J Periodontal Res 1997;32(6):487–96.
18. Sigusch B, Beier M, Klinger G, et al. A 2-step non-surgical procedure and systemic antibiotics in the treatment of rapidly progressive periodontitis. J Periodontol 2001;72(3):275–83.
19. Gomi K, Yashima A, Nagano T, et al. Effects of full-mouth scaling and root planing in conjunction with systemically administered azithromycin. J Periodontol 2007; 78(3):422–9.
20. Dastoor SF, Travan S, Neiva RF, et al. Effect of adjunctive systemic azithromycin with periodontal surgery in the treatment of chronic periodontitis in smokers: a pilot study. J Periodontol 2007;78(10):1887–96.
21. Cionca N, Giannopoulou C, Ugolotti G, et al. Amoxicillin and metronidazole as an adjunct to full-mouth scaling and root planing of chronic periodontitis. J Periodontol 2009;80(3):364–71.
22. Walker CB. The acquisition of antibiotic resistance in the periodontal microflora. Periodontol 2000 1996;10:79–88.
23. Bonito AJ, Lux L, Lohr KN. Impact of local adjuncts to scaling and root planing in periodontal disease therapy: a systematic review. J Periodontol 2005;76(8): 1227–36.
24. Goodson JM, Cugini MA, Kent RL, et al. Multicenter evaluation of tetracycline fiber therapy: II. Clinical response. J Periodontal Res 1991;26(4):371–9.
25. Garrett S, Johnson L, Drisko CH, et al. Two multi-center studies evaluating locally delivered doxycycline hyclate, placebo control, oral hygiene, and scaling and root planing in the treatment of periodontitis. J Periodontol 1999;70(5):490–503.
26. Wennstrom JL, Newman HN, MacNeill SR, et al. Utilisation of locally delivered doxycycline in non-surgical treatment of chronic periodontitis. A comparative multi-centre trial of 2 treatment approaches. J Clin Periodontol 2001;28(8): 753–61.
27. Machion L, Andia DC, Lecio G, et al. Locally delivered doxycycline as an adjunctive therapy to scaling and root planing in the treatment of smokers: a 2-year follow-up. J Periodontol 2006;77(4):606–13.
28. Williams RC, Paquette DW, Offenbacher S, et al. Treatment of periodontitis by local administration of minocycline microspheres: a controlled trial. J Periodontol 2001;72(11):1535–44.
29. Goodson JM, Gunsolley JC, Grossi SG, et al. Minocycline HCl microspheres reduce red-complex bacteria in periodontal disease therapy. J Periodontol 2007;78(8):1568–79.

30. Ainamo J, Lie T, Ellingsen BH, et al. Clinical responses to subgingival application of a metronidazole 25% gel compared to the effect of subgingival scaling in adult periodontitis. J Clin Periodontol 1992;19(9 Pt 2):723–9.
31. Pradeep AR, Sagar SV, Daisy H. Clinical and microbiologic effects of subgingivally delivered 0.5% azithromycin in the treatment of chronic periodontitis. J Periodontol 2008;79(11):2125–35.
32. Ciancio S. Non-surgical periodontal treatment. Proceedings of the World Workshop in Clinical Periodontics. 1989. p. II:II1–12.
33. Addy M. Oral hygiene products: potential for harm to oral and systemic health? Periodontol 2000 2008;48(1):54–65.
34. Fornell J, Sundin Y, Lindhe J. Effect of Listerine on dental plaque and gingivitis. Scand J Dent Res 1975;83(1):18–25.
35. DePaola LG, Overholser CD, Meiller TF, et al. Chemotherapeutic inhibition of supragingival dental plaque and gingivitis development. J Clin Periodontol 1989;16(5):311–5.
36. Gordon JM, Lamster IB, Seiger MC. Efficacy of Listerine antiseptic in inhibiting the development of plaque and gingivitis. J Clin Periodontol 1985;12(8):697–704.
37. Loe H, Schiott CR. The effect of mouthrinses and topical application of chlorhexidine on the development of dental plaque and gingivitis in man. J Periodontal Res 1970;5(2):79–83.
38. Flotra L, Gjermo P, Rolla G, et al. 4-Month study on the effect of chlorhexidine mouth washes on 50 soldiers. Scand J Dent Res 1972;80(1):10–7.
39. Overholser CD, Meiller TF, DePaola LG, et al. Comparative effects of 2 chemotherapeutic mouthrinses on the development of supragingival dental plaque and gingivitis. J Clin Periodontol 1990;17(8):575–9.
40. Kim YJ, Rossa C Jr, Kirkwood KL. Prostaglandin production by human gingival fibroblasts inhibited by triclosan in the presence of cetylpyridinium chloride. J Periodontol 2005;76(10):1735–42.
41. Pires JR, Rossa CJ, Pizzolitto AC. In vitro antimicrobial efficiency of a mouthwash containing Triclosan/Gantrez and sodium bicarbonate. Braz Oral Res 2007;21(4): 342–7.
42. Yazdankhah SP, Scheie AA, Hoiby EA, et al. Triclosan and antimicrobial resistance in bacteria: an overview. Microb Drug Resist 2006;12(2):83–90.
43. Walker C, Borden LC, Zambon JJ, et al. The effects of a 0.3% triclosan-containing dentifrice on the microbial composition of supragingival plaque. J Clin Periodontol 1994;21(5):334–41.
44. Jones CL, Ritchie JA, Marsh PD, et al. The effect of long-term use of a dentifrice containing zinc citrate and a non-ionic agent on the oral flora. J Dent Res 1988; 67(1):46–50.
45. Gusberti FA, Sampathkumar P, Siegrist BE, et al. Microbiological and clinical effects of chlorhexidine digluconate and hydrogen peroxide mouthrinses on developing plaque and gingivitis. J Clin Periodontol 1988;15(1):60–7.
46. Weitzman SA, Weitberg AB, Niederman R, et al. Chronic treatment with hydrogen peroxide. Is it safe? J Periodontol 1984;55(9):510–1.
47. Siegrist B, Gusberti F, Brecx M, et al. Efficacy of supervised rinsing with chlorhexidine digluconate in comparison to phenolic and plant alkaloid compounds. J Periodontal Res 1986;21(Suppl 16):60.
48. Offenbacher S. Periodontal diseases: pathogenesis. Ann Periodontol 1996;1(1): 821–78.
49. Greenwell H. Position paper. Guidelines for periodontal therapy. J Periodontol 2001;72(11):1624–8.

50. Reddy MS, Geurs NC, Gunsolley JC. Periodontal host modulation with antiprotei-nase, anti-inflammatory, and bone-sparing agents. A systematic review. Ann Periodontol 2003;8(1):12–37.
51. Birkedal-Hansen H. Role of cytokines and inflammatory mediators in tissue destruction. J Periodontal Res 1993;28(6 Pt 2):500–10.
52. Golub LM, Goodson JM, Lee HM, et al. Tetracyclines inhibit tissue collagenases. Effects of ingested low-dose and local delivery systems. J Periodontol 1985; 56(Suppl 11):93–7.
53. Burns FR, Stack MS, Gray RD, et al. Inhibition of purified collagenase from alkali-burned rabbit corneas. Invest Ophthalmol Vis Sci 1989;30(7):1569–75.
54. Golub LM, Ciancio S, Ramamamurthy NS, et al. Low-dose doxycycline therapy: effect on gingival and crevicular fluid collagenase activity in humans. J Periodontal Res 1990;25(6):321–30.
55. DeWitt DL, Meade EA, Smith WL. PGH synthase isoenzyme selectivity: the potential for safer nonsteroidal antiinflammatory drugs. Am J Med 1993;95(2A):40S–4S.
56. Dewhirst FE, Moss DE, Offenbacher S, et al. Levels of prostaglandin E2, thromboxane, and prostacyclin in periodontal tissues. J Periodontal Res 1983;18(2): 156–63.
57. Offenbacher S, Farr DH, Goodson JM. Measurement of prostaglandin E in crevicular fluid. J Clin Periodontol 1981;8(4):359–67.
58. Shimizu N, Ozawa Y, Yamaguchi M, et al. Induction of COX-2 expression by mechanical tension force in human periodontal ligament cells. J Periodontol 1998;69(6):670–7.
59. Holzhausen M, Rossa Junior C, Marcantonio Junior E, et al. Effect of selective cyclooxygenase-2 inhibition on the development of ligature-induced periodontitis in rats. J Periodontol 2002;73(9):1030–6.
60. Holzhausen M, Spolidorio DM, Muscara MN, et al. Protective effects of etoricoxib, a selective inhibitor of cyclooxygenase-2, in experimental periodontitis in rats. J Periodontal Res 2005;40(3):208–11.
61. Bezerra MM, de Lima V, Alencar VB, et al. Selective cyclooxygenase-2 inhibition prevents alveolar bone loss in experimental periodontitis in rats. J Periodontol 2000;71(6):1009–14.
62. Rogers MJ, Gordon S, Benford HL, et al. Cellular and molecular mechanisms of action of bisphosphonates. Cancer 2000;88(Suppl 12):2961–78.
63. Fleisch HA. Bisphosphonates: preclinical aspects and use in osteoporosis. Ann Med 1997;29(1):55–62.
64. Brunsvold MA, Chaves ES, Kornman KS, et al. Effects of a bisphosphonate on experimental periodontitis in monkeys. J Periodontol 1992;63(10):825–30.
65. Reddy MS, Weatherford TW 3rd, Smith CA, et al. Alendronate treatment of naturally-occurring periodontitis in beagle dogs. J Periodontol 1995;66(3): 211–7.
66. Rocha M, Nava LE, Vazquez de la Torre C, et al. Clinical and radiological improvement of periodontal disease in patients with type 2 diabetes mellitus treated with alendronate: a randomized, placebo-controlled trial. J Periodontol 2001;72(2):204–9.
67. Rocha ML, Malacara JM, Sanchez-Marin FJ, et al. Effect of alendronate on periodontal disease in postmenopausal women: a randomized placebo-controlled trial. J Periodontol 2004;75(12):1579–85.
68. Lane N, Armitage GC, Loomer P, et al. Bisphosphonate therapy improves the outcome of conventional periodontal treatment: results of a 12-month, randomized, placebo-controlled study. J Periodontol 2005;76(7):1113–22.

69. Jeffcoat MK, Cizza G, Shih WJ, et al. Efficacy of bisphosphonates for the control of alveolar bone loss in periodontitis. J Int Acad Periodontol 2007; 9(3):70–6.
70. El-Shinnawi UM, El-Tantawy SI. The effect of alendronate sodium on alveolar bone loss in periodontitis (clinical trial). J Int Acad Periodontol 2003;5(1):5–10.
71. Marx RE. Pamidronate (Aredia) and zoledronate (Zometa) induced avascular necrosis of the jaws: a growing epidemic. J Oral Maxillofac Surg 2003;61(9): 1115–7.
72. Ruggiero SL, Mehrotra B, Rosenberg TJ, et al. Osteonecrosis of the jaws associated with the use of bisphosphonates: a review of 63 cases. J Oral Maxillofac Surg 2004;62(5):527–34.
73. Odvina CV, Zerwekh JE, Rao DS, et al. Severely suppressed bone turnover: a potential complication of alendronate therapy. J Clin Endocrinol Metab 2005; 90(3):1294–301.
74. Caton JG, Ciancio SG, Blieden TM, et al. Subantimicrobial dose doxycycline as an adjunct to scaling and root planing: post-treatment effects. J Clin Periodontol 2001;28(8):782–9.
75. Gapski R, Barr JL, Sarment DP, et al. Effect of systemic matrix metalloproteinase inhibition on periodontal wound repair: a proof of concept trial. J Periodontol 2004;75(3):441–52.
76. Chang KM, Ryan ME, Golub LM, et al. Local and systemic factors in periodontal disease increase matrix-degrading enzyme activities in rat gingiva: effect of micocycline therapy. Res Commun Mol Pathol Pharmacol 1996; 91(3):303–18.
77. Novak MJ, Johns LP, Miller RC, et al. Adjunctive benefits of subantimicrobial dose doxycycline in the management of severe, generalized, chronic periodontitis. J Periodontol 2002;73(7):762–9.
78. Golub LM, McNamara TF, Ryan ME, et al. Adjunctive treatment with subantimicrobial doses of doxycycline: effects on gingival fluid collagenase activity and attachment loss in adult periodontitis. J Clin Periodontol 2001;28(2):146–56.
79. Assuma R, Oates T, Cochran D, et al. IL-1 and TNF antagonists inhibit the inflammatory response and bone loss in experimental periodontitis. J Immunol 1998; 160(1):403–9.
80. Graves DT, Delima AJ, Assuma R, et al. Interleukin-1 and tumor necrosis factor antagonists inhibit the progression of inflammatory cell infiltration toward alveolar bone in experimental periodontitis. J Periodontol 1998;69(12):1419–25.
81. Adams JL, Badger AM, Kumar S, et al. p38 MAP kinase: molecular target for the inhibition of pro-inflammatory cytokines. Prog Med Chem 2001;38:1–60.
82. Kumar S, Votta BJ, Rieman DJ, et al. IL-1- and TNF-induced bone resorption is mediated by p38 mitogen activated protein kinase. J Cell Physiol 2001;187(3): 294–303.
83. Rogers JE, Li F, Coatney DD, et al. A p38 mitogen-activated protein kinase inhibitor arrests active alveolar bone loss in a rat periodontitis model. J Periodontol 2007;78(10):1992–8.

Lasers and the Treatment of Chronic Periodontitis

Charles M. Cobb, DDS, MS, PhD[a],*, Samuel B. Low, DDS, MS[b],
Donald J. Coluzzi, DDS[c]

KEYWORDS

• Lasers • Periodontitis • Bacteria • Probing depth
• Clinical attachment level • Inflammation

For many intraoral soft-tissue surgical procedures the laser has become a desirable and dependable alternative to traditional scalpel surgery. The dental literature contains many case reports and uncontrolled case studies that report on the use of various laser wavelengths, predominantly diode, CO_2, Nd:YAG, Er:YAG, and Er, Cr:YSGG, for various intraoral soft-tissue procedures, such as frenectomy, gingivectomy and gingivoplasty, de-epithelization of reflected periodontal flaps, second stage exposure of dental implants, lesion ablation, incisional and excisional biopsies, irradiation of aphthous ulcers, removal of gingival pigmentation, and soft-tissue crown lengthening.[1-12] Lasers easily ablate and reshape oral soft tissues. In addition, lasers increase hemostasis through heat-induced coagulation and occlusion of arterioles, venules, and capillaries. The resulting hemostasis allows for a clear and fully visible surgical field. Because of the intense heat, lasers also have the advantage of a bactericidal effect at the target site. A few studies have reported that laser surgery, compared with traditional scalpel surgery, is less painful, features less swelling, and heals faster with less wound contraction.[13,14] However, there are conflicting opinions on pain and speed of wound healing. Several papers comparing lasers with traditional scalpel wounding have reported either an equivalent effect or that laser surgery is accompanied by more pain and slower healing.[15-19] The issues of pain and wound

This work was not funded by any agency or commercial enterprise and none of the authors has a conflict of interest that would compromise or affect on the manuscript content.
a Department of Periodontics, School of Dentistry, University of Missouri-Kansas City, 424 West 67th Terrace, Kansas City, MO 64113, USA
b Department of Periodontics, College of Dentistry, University of Florida, PO Box 100405, Gainesville, FL 32610-0405, USA
c Department of Preventive and Restorative Dental Sciences, University of California San Francisco School of Dentistry, 707 Parnassus Avenue, San Francisco, CA 94143-0758, USA
* Corresponding author.
E-mail address: cobbc@umkc.edu (C.M. Cobb).

Dent Clin N Am 54 (2010) 35–53
doi:10.1016/j.cden.2009.08.007
0011-8532/09/$ – see front matter © 2010 Elsevier Inc. All rights reserved.

healing, and wound contraction seem dependent on the judicious choice of parameters such as power, hertz, pulse duration, and time of exposure.[13]

Given the apparent usefulness of the laser, why, after almost 2 decades, does the use of dental lasers in periodontal therapy remain controversial? Is it because lasers challenge the traditional modalities of treating periodontitis or because of a lack of hard evidence on which to make an informed decision? One may argue in favor of one or both of these reasons. It is well known that many in private practice are using various types of lasers for the treatment of periodontal disease and most have expressed satisfaction with the results of therapy. However, several recent systematic reviews of the literature have suggested there is little evidence in support of the purported benefits of lasers in the treatment of periodontal disease compared with traditional periodontal therapy.[13,14,20–22] The obvious question then becomes, is the current use of dental laser for the treatment of periodontitis based on peer-reviewed published evidence obtained under controlled conditions or word-of-mouth, unconfirmed evidence?

A letter to the editor in a recent issue of the *Journal of Dental Education*[23] asked the following question: "Why is it that dentists are among the very few health professionals who can ignore critical evaluation of the scientific literature and treat patients with personal experience as its equal?" The authors suggest that many dentists may be providing treatment without critically evaluating whether such treatment is consistent with the best evidence.

The authors also present several possible reasons for ignoring the best available evidence, such as expediency, difficulty finding reliable evidence-based references, easy access to questionable information, and a desire for quick profits. Other reasons may include the introduction of new products without rigorous clinical trials. Regulatory agencies such as the US Food and Drug Administration (FDA) do not necessarily require clinical research before product marketing. As an example, in the case of dental lasers, the 510K FDA premarket notification process requires only that the applicant provide evidence that its device is substantially equivalent to 1 or more similar devices currently marketed in the US marketplace. A 510K premarket notification does not imply therapeutic equivalency or superiority. Indeed, the 510K process does not even require a clinical trial.[24]

Given the current conflicting opinions, this article presents the current peer-reviewed evidence on the use of dental lasers for the treatment of chronic periodontitis.

WAVELENGTH

Wavelength can be related to collateral tissue damage. In general, the shorter wavelength lasers (eg, 809 nm to 980 nm diodes and 1064 nm Nd:YAG) are more likely to penetrate deeper into soft tissues.[4,5] The extent of tissue penetration by shorter wavelengths is related to their affinity for pigmented tissues and a low absorption coefficient in water. The potential for undesired tissue penetration can be controlled with proper selection of parameters, such as power level, pulse repetition rate, pulse width, and energy density. In contrast, the longer wavelengths (2940 nm Er:YAG, 2780 nm Er, Cr:YSGG, and 10,600 nm CO_2) show comparatively more shallow tissue penetration because of their high absorption coefficients in water.[4,5] To avoid unintended consequences, the least amount of power required to achieve the desired clinical result should be chosen. Hard tissues and periosteum subjacent to thin oral mucosa (thin biotype), the gingival margin, or gingiva overlying prominent roots, are particularly vulnerable to thermal insult (**Fig. 1A–D**). The potential for damage to dental hard

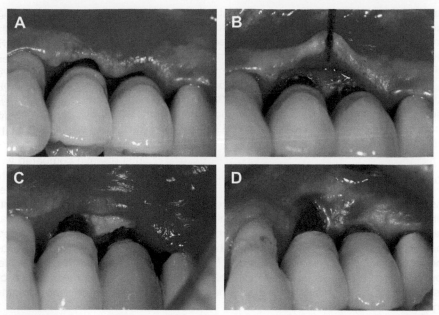

Fig. 1. Interproximal soft-tissue cratering with underlying bone necrosis around 2 dental implants following laser treatment of periimplantitis using inappropriate energy density and duration of exposure. Photos in sequence: (*A, B*) 1 month post laser treatment; (*C*) sequestration of necrotic interproximal and facial bone at 2 months post treatment; and (*D*) healing at 3 months post treatment. (Patient referred to and photos taken by Keigm Crook, DDS, Albuquerque, NM.)

tissues results from uncontrolled penetration during soft-tissue procedures that, in turn, results from improper choice of parameters while using a short wavelength laser or the conductive heat effects arising from superheating of char produced by longer wavelengths.[5] Moreover, only the erbium family of lasers have a specific indication for use on dental hard tissue, and other wavelengths should be avoided. The clinician is well advised to assess tissue thickness before initiating any laser procedure involving the gingival sulcus or the periodontal pocket area.

LASERS AND PERIODONTAL THERAPY

As a basic premise, it should be understood that the gold standard for successful treatment of chronic periodontitis is gain in clinical attachment level.[13,25] However, other clinical goals are often considered as creditable end-points and should be considered, such as maintenance of esthetics, complete debridement of root surface accretions, regeneration of bone, periodontal ligament and cementum, and patient preference.

Basic knowledge and understanding of the pathogenesis of plaque-induced periodontal disease continues to evolve.[26–29] The current model for plaque-induced periodontal diseases includes the initial microbial challenge, a subsequent host inflammatory response, and various risk factors that contribute to host susceptibility and progression of the disease.[26–29] Considering the microbial component, it seems logical that laser irradiation with its bactericidal effect would have significant potential as an alternative or adjunct to traditional nonsurgical therapy (ie, scaling and root planing). All dental lasers have a thermal effect. In general, most nonsporulating bacteria, including periodontopathic anaerobes, are readily deactivated at temperatures of 50°C.[30] Coagulation of the inflamed soft-tissue wall of a periodontal pocket and hemostasis are both achieved at a temperature of 60°C.[31]

Over the last decade, various dental laser wavelengths have been used by clinicians in the treatment of periodontitis, most commonly the diode lasers (809–980 nm), Nd:YAG (1064 nm), Er:YAG and Er,Cr:YSGG (2940 nm and 2780 nm, respectively), and the CO_2 (10,600 nm). In addition, photodynamic therapy protocols use diode lasers with wavelengths in the range of 635 nm to 690 nm combined with a photosensitizer to eradicate subgingival microbes.

ND:YAG LASER

Laser-mediated periodontal therapy is based on the purported benefits derived from subgingival soft-tissue curettage and significant decreases in subgingival bacterial loads. **Table 1** seems to indicate that Nd:YAG lasers are used primarily for these specific reasons, that is, laser-assisted subgingival soft-tissue curettage and reduction of subgingival microbial populations.[32-41] The exception is the laser-assisted new attachment procedure (LANAP)[39] which purports to promote regeneration of lost periodontal support structures (eg, cementum, periodontal ligament, and supporting alveolar bone).

Despite the increasing use of the Nd:YAG laser for treating periodontitis, well-designed and adequately powered studies (eg, that include enough subjects to see a difference if one exists) are severely limited and the overall quality of the body of evidence is insufficient to support evidence-based decision making. For various reasons performing a meta-analysis using data from existing clinical trials that have used the Nd:YAG laser as the test therapy is not possible. In fact, one can legitimately argue that deriving evidence-based conclusions from the published literature is overtly speculative as the body of evidence is weak and often confusing. For example, in the outcomes measurement of periodontal probing depth (PPD) in the clinical trials listed in **Table 1**, 2 studies did not measure PPD as an end-point[32,35]; 1 study did not provide data for PPD measurements[41]; 3 studies reported little or no difference in PPD reduction when comparing laser-treated sites with control sites[36-38]; 1 study reported a greater mean decrease in PPD in the control group (scaling and root planing, ie, SRP) than in the laser-treated group[33]; 1 study reported the laser improved PPD compared with untreated controls[34]; 1 study reported a decrease in PPD when the laser was used in combination with locally delivered minocycline and compared with a sham procedure[40]; and 1 study reported the laser improved PPD compared with historic controls (ie, data reported in other studies used for comparison).[39] This latter study[39] reported large standard deviations for mean PPD reductions in laser-treated pockets, indicating either a significant variation in technique or a significant degree of unpredictability in the procedure.

Other examples of inconsistencies in reporting of treatment outcomes are also seen in **Table 1**. Only 3[34,38,40] of the 10 studies measured gains in clinical attachment levels (CAL), despite the fact that CAL is considered the gold standard for demonstrating effect of periodontal therapy. Six of the 10 studies reported bleeding on probing (BOP) as an outcome although, similar to probing depth (PD), there was considerable variability in results. Five of the 10 studies did not measure reductions in subgingival microbial populations and of the 5 studies that did report on this parameter, 3 showed no significant difference,[32,36,41] 1 favored the SRP control group,[33] and 1 favored the laser-treated group[34] although no data were presented.

Although calculating the average of a series of means is risky at best and not a reliable statistical method, it does allow trends to be viewed. Given this caveat, **Table 1** shows a difference in PD reduction between laser treatment groups and controls of 0.09 mm, a gain in CAL of 0.33 mm (favoring the Nd:YAG laser) and essentially no difference in reductions in BOP or subgingival microbial loads.

Probably as a result of the nonsurgical character attributed to laser periodontal therapy, most clinical studies comparing the laser to standard therapy in the treatment of periodontitis use SRP as the control rather than conventional surgical procedures. The concept of regeneration of the periodontal attachment apparatus as an ultimate goal is, in many cases, more of an ideal than a pragmatic achievement. The debate will continue over regenerated connective tissue attachment versus long-junctional epithelial attachment, the latter often the result of many surgical and nonsurgical periodontal procedures.[42,43] However, for purposes of comparison, it would seem that laser procedures may have a positive adjunctive effect on periodontal regeneration by decreasing bacteria, producing an etching effect on root surfaces, removing granulation tissue, and de-epithelialization of the pocket soft-tissue wall. When laser therapies are compared with conventional open-flap procedures, with or without the addition of biologic mediators such as enamel matrix protein derivatives, the conclusions are consistent in that no statistical or clinically significant differences have been reported when comparing traditional surgery with laser-mediated periodontal surgery.[44,45]

A recent human histologic study using the Nd:YAG laser in a specific protocol, the LANAP, reports new cementum and new connective tissue attachment on previously diseased root surfaces, and bone regeneration.[46] By contrast, the SRP controls exhibited repair via a long-junctional epithelium with no evidence of bone regeneration. Moreover, there were no adverse changes associated with the laser group.

Several issues concerning this study are worthy of consideration. First, the study was not blinded. Second, the study is basically a proof of principle study as the number of specimens is quite small (ie, 6 pairs of single-rooted teeth). The limited number of specimens severely restricts extrapolation of results to the general population. Third, the study used pretreatment notches in the teeth as histologic reference points. Such notches are difficult to place subgingivally and, therefore, it is hard to determine the site of placement, and difficult to detect on histologic specimens that have been demineralized for sectioning. Fourth, the study did not use stents to aid clinical measurement. Consequently, given that manual probing is susceptible to variation, the results achieved fall within the range of acceptable measurement error for PPD and CAL of ±1 mm reported by other clinical trials devoted to measuring such parameters.[47,48] Thus, it can justifiably be argued that the reported gain in CAL and reduction in PD may only equal that achieved by SRP. Fifth, the materials and methods are vague: "Sections were cut in 200 micron increments until the notch was found, then serially sectioned at 200 micron increments (7 micron thick sections) until the notch was no longer visible. The 3 most central sections were then sent ... for evaluation." Depending on interpretation, the "3 most central sections" can represent either 3.2% or 30% of the total possible number of 7 μm sections. Regardless of the interpretation, the resulting number of sections represents a limited histologic assessment and says nothing about consistency of effect across the depth and width of the treated defect. Lastly, all treated teeth were single-rooted. Thus, no conclusions can be made regarding the effect of treatment on multirooted teeth presenting with furcation involvement. The ultimate test of the regenerative powers of the LANAP protocol would be regeneration of horizontal bone loss, a study yet to be done.

Table 1
Summary of clinical trials for Nd:YAG laser treatment of periodontitis (4–6 mm PDs)

Reference	No. of Subjects, Length of Study	Reduction in PPD (mm): Laser vs Control	Gain in CAL (mm): Laser vs Control	Reduction in BOP (%): Laser vs Control	Reduction in Microbes	Comment
Ben Hatit et al, 1996[32]	14, 70 d	n.a.	n.a.	n.a.	No significant difference	Treatment groups: laser used at different energy densities vs SRP (control)
Radvar et al, 1996[33]	11, 42 d	0.50 vs 1.70	n.a.	10 vs 45	SRP	Treatment groups: laser vs SRP (control)
Neill & Mellonig, 1997[34]	10, 180d	1.30 vs 0.40	1.10 vs 1.00	Yes	Laser	Treatment groups: laser vs SRP vs untreated control
Liu et al, 1999[35]	8, 84 d	n.a.	n.a.	n.a.	n.a.	Treatment groups: laser vs SRP vs laser + SRP vs SRP + laser. Outcome measure was level of IL-1β in GCF
Gutknecht et al, 2002[36]	20, 175d	0.85 vs 0.80	n.a.	85 vs 75	No significant difference	Treatment groups: SRP+laser once/wk for 3 weeks vs SRP vs untreated control
Sjostrom et al,[a] 2002[37]	27, 120d	1.40 vs 1.40	n.a.	27 vs 29	n.a.	Treatment groups: laser+SRP+laser vs SRP (control)
Miyazaki et al, 2003[38]	18, 84 d	1.43 vs 1.36	0.50 vs 0.57	43 vs 34	n.a.	Treatment groups: Nd:YAG laser vs CO$_2$ laser vs ultrasonic scaling (control)

Harris et al, 2004[39]	75,[b] 180d	1.55 vs 1.29	n.a.	n.a.	n.a.	Treatment groups: LANAP protocol vs historic controls
Noguchi et al, 2005[40]	16, 90 d	1.57 vs n.a.	1.52 vs n.a.	63 vs n.a.	n.a.	Treatment groups: laser vs laser + local minocycline vs laser + povidone-iodine irrigation vs sham laser control
Verhagen et al, 2006[41]	15, 90 d	No significant difference (no data given)	n.a.	16 vs 17	No significant difference	Treatment groups: SRP + laser with and without systemic antibiotics vs SRP with and without systemic antibiotics. Use of antibiotics had no impact on parameter outcomes
Average Difference: laser vs control		1.23 vs 1.14 0.09	1.04 vs 0.71 0.33	41 vs 40 1	1 favored laser 1 favored SRP 3 no significant difference 5 studies n.a.	

All numbers for reductions in PD and BOP and gains in CAL represent means.

Abbreviation: n.a., did not measure parameter.

[a] Nd:YCG (1061 nm).

[b] Includes 10 patients from Neill and Mellonig's study.[34]

Table 2

Summary of clinical trials for Er:YAG/Er,Cr:YSGG laser treatment of periodontitis (4–6 mm PDs)

Reference	No. of Subjects, Length of Study	Reduction in PPD (mm): Laser vs Control	Gain in CAL (mm): Laser vs Control	Reduction in BOP (%): Laser vs Control	Reduction in Microbes	Comment
Schwarz et al, 2001[59]	20, 180 d	2.00 vs 1.60	1.90 vs 1.00	77 vs 56	No significant difference	Treatment groups: laser vs SRP (control)
Schwarz et al, 2003[60]	20, 1 y	2.00 vs n.a.	1.60 vs n.a.	16 vs n.a.	No significant difference	Treatment groups: laser+SRP vs laser (control)
Schwarz et al,[a] 2003[61]	20, 2 y	1.60 vs 1.30	1.40 vs 0.70	64 vs 46	No significant difference	Article reports long-term results of the Schwarz, et al, 2001 study[59]
Schwarz et al, 2003[44]	22, 180 d	4.00 vs 4.10	3.20 vs 3.30	35 vs 26	n.a.	Treatment groups: access flap surgery + laser debridement + enamel matrix protein derivative (test) vs access flap surgery + SRP + enamel matrix protein derivative (control)
Sculean et al, 2004[45]	23, 180 d	1.52 vs 1.57	1.11 vs 1.11	23 vs 31	n.a.	Treatment groups: laser vs flap surgery and debridement of root and defect (control)
Sculean et al, 2004[62]	20, 180 d	3.70 vs 3.20	2.60 vs 1.50	63 vs 59	n.a.	Treatment groups: laser vs ultrasonic scaling (control)
Tomasi et al, 2006[63]	20, 120 d	1.10 vs 1.00	0.60 vs 0.40	40 vs 40	No significant difference	Treatment groups: laser vs ultrasonic scaler (control)

Crespi et al,[b] 2007[64]	25, 2 y	2.88 vs 1.00	2.92 vs 1.32	n.a.	n.a.	Treatment groups: laser vs ultrasonic scaler (control). Treated 5–6 mm $\geq$ 7 mm PDs
Gaspirc & Skaleric, 2007[65]	25, 5 y	2.79 vs 2.87	1.72 vs 1.76	39 vs 23	n.a.	Treatment groups: laser + surgery vs modified Widman flap (control)
Kelbauskiene et al, 2007[66]	10, 84 d	2.00 vs 0.97	n.a.	68 vs 60	n.a.	Treatment groups: laser vs SRP clinical trial using Er,Cr:YSGG laser
Lopes et al,[c] 2008[67]	21, 30 d	1.60 vs 1.67 (L+SRP vs SRP)	0.21 vs 0.48 (L+SRP vs SRP)	n.a.	n.a.	Treatment groups: laser + SRP vs laser vs SRP vs untreated control
Average of the mean		2.29 vs 1.93	1.73 vs 1.23	47 vs 43	4 no significant difference	
Difference: laser vs control		0.36	0.45	4	7 studies n.a.	

All numbers for reductions in PD and BOP and gains in CAL represent means.

Abbreviation: n.a., did not measure parameter.

[a] Paper reports the long-term results of the Schwarz et al, 2001 study.[59]

[b] Treated 5–6 mm and 7 mm PD.

[c] Treated 5–9 mm PD. Mean PD for all Tx groups ranged from 6.28 to 6.87 mm.

Table 3
Summary of clinical trials for diode laser treatment of periodontitis (4–6 mm PDs)

References	No. of Subjects, Length of Study	Reduction in PPD (mm) Laser vs Control	Gain in CAL (mm) Laser vs Control	Reduction in BOP (%) Laser vs Control	Reduction in Microbes	Comment
Moritz et al, 1998[68]	50, 180 d	1.30 vs 0.40	n.a.	97 vs 67[a]	No significant difference	Treatment groups: scaling + laser at 1, 8, and 16 weeks vs scaling + H_2O_2 (control) rinsing at 1, 8, and 16 weeks
Borrajo et al, 2004[69]	30, 42 d	n.a.	0.81 vs 0.85	72 vs 53	n.a.	Treatment groups: SRP + laser vs SRP (control)
Qadri et al, 2005[70]	17, 42 d	0.90 vs 0.20	n.a.	n.a.	No significant difference	Treatment groups: laser vs laser sham (control). Measured GCF levels of IL-1β and MMP-8 and reported no significant difference between groups
Kreisler et al, 2005[71]	22, 90 d	1.8 vs 1.6		38 vs 34	n.a.	Treatment groups: all patients received SRP. Subsequently, 2 quadrants in each patient were treated with the laser
Kamma et al, 2006[72]	30, 84 d	Laser 2.00 SRP 2.34 L+SRP 2.80 Control 0.13	Laser 1.94 SRP 1.87 L+SRP 2.14 Control 0.27	Laser 65 SRP 57 L+SRP 63 Control 61	Laser	Treatment groups: laser vs SRP vs laser + SRP vs untreated control. Aggressive periodontitis with clinical attachment loss of $\geq$ 5 mm
Average of the means		1.7 vs 1.14	1.52 vs 1.34	58 vs 53	1 favored laser	
L+SRP vs SRP					2 no significant difference	
Difference: L+SRP vs SRP		0.56	0.18	15	2 studies n.a.	

All numbers for reductions in PD and BOP and gains in CAL represent means.

Abbreviation: n.a., did not measure parameter.

[a] Percent of sites showing improvement.

With respect to laser-mediated periodontal regeneration, in a study by Schwartz and colleagues[49] beagle dogs with naturally occurring periodontitis were treated with an Er:YAG laser; ultrasonic scaling was used as a control. Both treatment groups exhibited new cementum formation with embedded collagen fibers. The investigators concluded that both therapies supported the formation of new connective tissue attachment.

The Nd:YAG laser is absorbed selectively by certain pigments, including melanin and hemoglobin. Given this selective absorption in darker pigments, proponents of this wavelength have promoted the laser as being effective against the pigmented bacteria frequently associated with periodontal diseases, eg, *Porphyromonas* spp, *Prevotella* spp, *Tannerella* spp. However, the common periodontal diseases exhibit a subgingival biofilm comprised of a diverse population of bacteria, most of which are not pigment producers.[50]

ER:YAG AND ER,CR:YSGG LASERS

Two different wavelengths of erbium lasers are currently available for clinical use: the Er:YAG (2940 nm) and the Er,Cr:YSGG (2780 nm). Each system ablates soft and hard tissues with minimal heat-related side effects. It has been suggested that the erbium wavelengths present the broadest range of application for clinical dentistry and are likely the most suitable lasers for periodontal therapy.[13,21,51,52]

The erbium lasers are effective in removing calculus and reducing PPD. Several studies have demonstrated safe and effective root substance removal without negative thermal effects, comparable with conventional instrumentation.[53–55] Not surprisingly, these lasers are bactericidal against in vitro cultures of *Porphyromonas gingivalis* and *Aggregatibacter* (formally *Actinobacillus*) *actinomycetemcomitans*,[56] and effective in removing absorbed root surface endotoxins.[57,58]

In **Table 2**, a collective average for the 11 clinical trials shows equivalent or slightly greater reductions in PPD (2.29 mm vs 1.93 mm), gains in CAL (1.73 vs 1.26 mm), and decreased BOP (47% vs 43%) when comparing laser therapy with the control treatments.[44,45,59–67] The one paradoxic exception is that of the 4 studies reporting the effect of treatment on subgingival microbial levels; none showed a significant difference between treatment groups.[59–61,63]

Three of the clinical trials deviated from the usual design in that they either combined the Er:YAG laser with flap surgery, with and without adjunctive use of enamel matrix protein,[44] compared the laser with traditional access flap surgery,[45] or compared the laser with the modified Widman flap.[65] For PPD reduction and gains in CAL the results were essentially equivalent.

DIODE LASER

The most widely used lasers in the diode family are the gallium-aluminum-arsenide (GaAlAs) laser (810 nm) and the indium-gallium-arsenide (InGaAs) laser (980 nm). A low initial investment cost and ease of use by dental hygienists are undoubtedly major factors for this popularity. Thus, given the apparent widespread use of the diode for treatment of slight to moderate periodontitis, it is surprising to realize that currently there are only 5 published clinical trials (**Table 3**). As with the Nd:YAG laser, the purported benefits of diode laser periodontal therapy are based on the premise that subgingival curettage is an effective treatment and that significant reduction in subgingival microbial populations are predictably achieved.

The 5 studies[68–72] presented in **Table 3** used various control groups with which to compare diode laser therapy. In 4 studies,[68,69,71,72] the diode laser was used

Table 4
Summary of clinical trials for photodynamic therapy (PDT) using a diode laser plus a photosensitizer for the treatment of periodontitis pockets with 4–6 mm probing depths

Reference	Laser Type and Photosensitizer	No. of Subjects, Length of Study	Reduction in PPD (mm): PDT vs SRP	Gain in CAL (mm): PDT vs SRP	Reduction in BOP (%): PDT vs SRP	Reduction in Microbes	Comment
Yilmaz et al, 2002[80]	Diode (685 nm); Methylene Blue	1032, d	PDT + SRP 0.66 / PDT 0.23 / SRP 0.49 / OHI 0.19	n.a.	PDT + SRP 60 / PDT 17 / SRP 50 / OHI 20	No significant difference	Treatment groups: laser + SRP vs laser vs SRP vs OHI (control). Photosensitizer used in both laser groups
Andersen et al, 2007[81]	Diode (670 nm); Methylene Blue	33, 84 d	PDT+ SRP 1.11 / PDT 0.67 / SRP 0.74	PDT+ SRP 0.62 / PDT 0.14 / SRP 0.36	PDT+SRP 73 / SRP 56	n.a.	Treatment groups: PDT + SRP vs PDT vs SRP
de Oliveira et al, 2007[82]	Diode (690 nm); Phenothiazine	10, 90 d	PDT+SRP 1.43 / SRP 0.94	PDT + SRP 1.19 / SRP 1.52 (relative clinical attachment level)	PDT+ SRP 38 / SRP 39	n.a.	Treatment groups: PDT vs SRP (control). Mean PD was 4.92 mm in aggressive periodontitis
Braun et al, 2008[83]	Diode (660 nm); Phenothiazine	20, 90 d	PDT+SRP 0.8 / SRP 0.7	n.a.	PDT+SRP 56 / SRP 51	n.a.	Treatment groups: PDT + SRP vs SRP (control)
de Oliveira et al, 2009[84]	Diode (660 nm); Phenothiazine	10, 90 d	n.a.	n.a.	n.a.	n.a.	Treatment groups: PDT + SRP vs SRP (control). No significant difference in GCF levels of TNF-α or RANKL
Polansky et al 2009[85]	Diode (680 nm); HELBO blue	58, 90 d	PDT+SRP 1.24 / SRP 1.03	PDT+SRP 0.91	PDT+SRP 53 / SRP 41	No significant difference	Treatment groups: PDT+SRP vs SRP (control)
Average of the means PDT+SRP vs SRP			PDT+SRP 1.05 / SRP 0.78	PDT+SRP 0.94 / SRP 0.94	PDT+SRP 56 / SRP 47		
Difference: PDT+SRP vs SRP			0.27	0.03	9		

All numbers for reductions in PD and BOP and gains in CAL represent means.
Abbreviations: n.a., did not measure parameter; OHI, oral hygiene index.

Table 5
Comparative summary of results from clinical trials using Nd:YAG, Er:YAG, or diode lasers
for treatment of periodontal (4–6 mm PDs)

LaserType (Number of ClinicalTrials)	Reduction in PPD (mm)	Gain in CAL (mm)	Reduction in BOP (%)	Reduction in Microbes
Nd:YAG (n = 10)	1.23	1.04	41	2/10[a]
Er:YAG/Er,Cr:YSGG (n = 11)	2.30	1.68	47	0/11
Diode (n = 5)	1.70	1.52	68	1/5[b]
Photodynamic therapy (n =5)	1.05	0.91	56	0/5

[a] 1 study favored the laser and 1 study favored SRP.
[b] 1 study favored the laser.

adjunctively with SRP. Control groups consisted of SRP in 2 studies,[69,71] a sham laser treatment in 1 study,[70] and an initial scaling followed by periodic hydrogen peroxide or saline oral rinses in the remaining 2 studies.[68,71] None of the studies measured all 4 of the usual clinical parameters, that is, reductions in PPD, BOP, and subgingival microbes, or gains in CAL. Consequently, given the limited number of studies and the diversity in experimental design, it is not possible to combine the 5 studies for the purpose of a meta-analysis.

Despite these limitations it is possible to discern trends. For example, as noted in **Table 3**, when comparing the laser treatment groups with their specific controls, the laser groups showed greater reductions in PPD (1.70 mm vs 1.14 mm) and BOP (68% vs 53%) but a nearly equivalent gain in CAL (1.52 mm vs 1.34 mm). Three of the 5 studies measured reductions in microbes but only 1[72] reported a significant difference that favored the laser. The remaining 2 studies reported no significant differences between treatment groups.[68,70] Despite the equivalency between laser-treated sites versus controls, uncontrolled case studies continue to report successful periodontal therapy when using the diode and Nd:YAG lasers as adjuncts to SRP.

Diode lasers are effective for soft-tissue applications, offering excellent incision, hemostasis, and coagulation.[73] However, diode wavelengths when combined with the appropriate choice of parameters can result in penetration of soft tissues ranging from about 0.5 mm to 3 mm.[14] Thus, 1 must select parameters with caution to avoid undesired collateral damage. In this regard, the diode and Nd:YAG lasers are contraindicated for calculus removal. They both exhibit poor energy absorption in mineralized tissues and thus offer the possibility of excessive generation of heat caused by their interaction with darkly colored deposits. However, given the current recommended parameters, the possibility of inducing root surface damage is virtually impossible.[74,75]

PHOTODYNAMIC THERAPY

Photodynamic therapy (PDT) involves the combination of visible light, usually using a low wavelength diode laser (635 nm to 690 nm) and a photosensitizer. The photosensitizer is generally an organic dye or similar compound capable of absorbing light of a specific wavelength, after which it is transformed from a ground singlet state to a longer-lived excited triplet state.[76] The longer lifetime of the triplet state enables the interaction of the excited photosensitizer with the surrounding tissue molecules. It is generally accepted that the generation of the cytotoxic species produced during

PDT occurs while in the triplet state.[77,78] The cytotoxic product, generally O_2, cannot migrate more than 0.02 μm after this formation, thus making it ideal for the local application of PDT without endangering distant biomolecules, cells, or organs.[79]

As with the diode laser, there are a relatively small number of published clinical trials.[80–84] Given the apparent potential for PDT, it is discouraging that the collective differences reported for measurable clinical parameters are not particularly noteworthy (Table 4). The aggregate of clinical trials shows a reduction in PPD for PDT versus SRP of 1.0 mm versus 0.72 mm, respectively. Reduction in BOP was somewhat better: 57% for PDT versus 49% for SRP. Gains in CAL were nearly equal, 0.91 mm for PDT versus 0.94 mm for SRP. The major reason for using PDT is to effect reductions in subgingival microbes. Thus, it is surprising that only 1 of the 5 published clinical trials measured this parameter[80] and that study reported no significant difference between PDT and SRP treatment groups. In addition, de Oliveira and colleagues[84] compared treatment of aggressive periodontitis with PDT versus SRP and reported no significant differences between treatment groups for measures of gingival crevicular fluid (GCF) levels of tumor necrosis factor-alpha (TNF-α) or nuclear factor-kappa B ligand (RANKL), both factors being involved in bone resorption.

CO_2 LASER

The carbon dioxide wavelength is effective in removing soft tissue and inflamed pocket tissues while achieving good hemostasis. However, there are only 2 published clinical trials showing the effect of this wavelength on PD.[38] One study compared the Nd:YAG with ultrasonic scaling and the CO_2 laser and reported no significant difference between the 3 treatments. Choi and colleagues[86] measured changes in GCF levels of interleukin-1beta (IL-1β) at 6 weeks and PPD, BOP, and CAL at 6 months following treatment of periodontitis by traditional flap surgery versus flap surgery plus CO_2 laser irradiation of the exposed root surfaces using 2 different energy densities. The investigators reported no significant differences between treatment groups for reduced PPD (flap + laser groups, 2.7 mm vs flap surgery alone, 2.2 mm) and reduction in BOP (flap + laser groups, 61% vs flap surgery alone, 69%). Paradoxically, CAL gains were statistically significantly better for 1 of the CO_2 treatment groups, as were reductions in IL-1β. The primary caution when using the CO_2 laser for subgingival periodontal therapy relates to the wavelength's high absorption by hydroxyapatite and water. The clinician is well advised to carefully direct the energy beam and use low powers and low energy densities to avoid damage to healthy hard tissues. The recently introduced super-pulse mode reduces the potential for adverse effects caused by excessive heat generation during interaction with hard tissues.

SUMMARY

Many questions remain to be answered on use of lasers as a singular modality or as an adjunct for the treatment of periodontitis. Although the adjunctive use of lasers with traditional treatment modalities is less controversial, published clinical trials indicate only a slightly greater benefit should be expected with respect to gains in CAL and reductions in PPD, BOP, and subgingival microbial loads (Table 5). A recent publication noted that a meta-analysis of clinical trials was impossible because of the lack of homogeneity between studies.[21] Although the collective evidence was considered weak, the investigators did note that Er:YAG laser monotherapy resulted in similar clinical outcomes compared with SRP for up to 24 months post treatment.[21] Clearly, additional well-designed randomized, blinded, controlled longitudinal studies are necessary to provide clear and meaningful evidence to validate the use of this technology in periodontal therapy. Because of the current lack of published well-designed clinical trials, clinicians using lasers for the treatment of periodontitis must be cognizant of safety issues and should expect limited clinical improvement in periodontal status.

REFERENCES

1. Haytac MC, Ustun Y, Esen E, et al. Combined treatment approach of gingivectomy and CO_2 laser for cyclosporine-induced gingival overgrowth. Quintessence Int 2007;38(1):e54–9.
2. Gontijo I, Navarro RS, Haypek P, et al. The applications of diode and Er:YAG lasers in labial frenectomy in infant patients. J Dent Child 2005;72(1):10–5.
3. Fiorotti RC, Bertonlini MM, Nicola JH, et al. Early lingual frenectomy assisted by CO_2 laser helps prevention and treatment of functional alterations caused by ankyloglossia. Int J Orofacial Myology 2004;30:64–71.
4. Parker S. Lasers and soft tissue: 'loose' soft tissue surgery. Br Dent J 2007;202(4): 185–91.
5. Parker S. Lasers and soft tissue: 'fixed' soft tissue surgery. Br Dent J 2007;202(5): 247–53.
6. Bornstein MM, Winzap-Kalin C, Cochran DL, et al. The CO_2 laser for excisional biopsies of oral lesions: a case series study. Int J Periodontics Restorative Dent 2005;25(3):221–9.
7. Bladowski M, Konarska-Choroszucha H, Choroszucha T. Comparison of treatment results of recurrent aphthous stomatitis (RAS) with low- and high-power laser irradiation vs. a pharmaceutical method (5-year study). J Oral Laser Appl 2004;4(3):191–209.
8. Esen E, Haytac MC, Oz IA, et al. Gingival melanin pigmentation and its treatment with the CO2 laser. Oral Surg Oral Med Oral Pathol Oral Radiol Endod 2004;98(5): 522–7.
9. Israel M, Rossmann JA. An epithelial exclusion technique using the CO_2 laser for the treatment of periodontal defects. Compend Cont Ed Dent 1998;19(1):86–8, 90, 92–5.
10. Centty IG, Blank LW, Levy BA, et al. Carbon dioxide laser for de-epithelialization of periodontal flaps. J Periodontol 1997;68(8):763–9.
11. Arnabat-Dominguez J, Espana-Tost AJ, Berini-Aytes L, et al. Erbium:YAG laser application in the second phase of implant surgery: a pilot study in 20 patients. Int J Oral Maxillofac Implants 2003;18(1):104–12.
12. Lee EA. Laser-assisted crown lengthening procedures in the esthetic zone: contemporary guidelines and techniques. Contemp Esthetics 2007;11(3):36–42.
13. Cobb CM. Lasers in periodontics: a review of the literature. J Periodontol 2006; 77(4):545–64.
14. Aoki A, Mizutani K, Takasaki AA, et al. Current status of clinical laser applications in periodontal therapy. Gen Dent 2008;56(7):674–87.
15. Strauss RA, et al. A comparison of postoperative pain parameters between CO_2 laser and scalpel biopsies. J Oral Laser Appl 2006;6(1):39–42.
16. Lippert BM, Teymoortash A, Folz BJ, et al. Wound healing after laser treatment of oral and oropharyngeal cancer. Lasers Med Sci 2003;18(1):36–42.
17. Arashiro DS, Rapley JW, Cobb CM, et al. Histologic evaluation of porcine skin incisions produced by CO_2 laser, electrosurgery and scalpel. Int J Periodontics Restorative Dent 1996;16(5):479–91.

18. Williams TM, Cobb CM, Rapley JW, et al. Histologic evaluation of alveolar bone following CO_2 laser removal of connective tissue from periodontal defects. Int J Periodontics Restorative Dent 1995;15(5):497–506.
19. Romanos GE, Pelekanos S, Strub JR. A comparative histologic study of wound healing following Nd:YAG laser with different energy parameters and conventional surgical incision in rat skin. J Clin Laser Med Surg 1995;13(1):11–6.
20. Karlsson MR, Löfgren CID, Jansson HM. The effect of laser therapy as an adjunct to non-surgical periodontal treatment in subjects with chronic periodontitis: a systematic review. J Periodontol 2008;79(11):2021–8.
21. Schwarz F, Aoki A, Becker J, et al. Laser application in non-surgical periodontal therapy: a systematic review. J Clin Periodontol 2008;35(Suppl 8):29–44.
22. Slot DE, Kranendonk A, Paraskevas S, et al. The effect of a pulsed Nd:YAG laser in non-surgical periodontal therapy: a systematic review. J Periodontol 2009; 80(7):1041–56.
23. Spielman AI, Wolff MS. Letter to the editor: overcoming barriers to implementing evidence-based dentistry. J Dent Educ 2008;72(2):263–4.
24. US Food and Drug Administration. Premarket notification 510(k). Available at: http://www.fda.gov/CDRH/DEVADVICE/314.html. Accessed March 1, 2009.
25. Cobb CM. Non-surgical pocket therapy: mechanical. Ann Periodontol 1996;1(1): 443–90.
26. Van Dyke TE. Cellular and molecular susceptibility determinants for periodontitis. Periodontol 2000. 2007;45:10–3.
27. Kinane DF, Bartold MP. Clinical relevance of the host responses of periodontitis. Periodontol 2000. 2007;43:278–93.
28. Yoshie H, Kobayashi T, Tai H, et al. The role of genetic polymorphisms in periodontitis. Periodontol 2000. 2007;43:102–32.
29. Haffajee AD, Socransky SS. Introduction to microbial aspects of periodontal biofilm communities, development and treatment. Periodontol 2000. 2006;42:7–12.
30. Russell AD. Lethal effects of heat on bacterial physiology and structure. Sci Prog 2003;86(1–2):115–37.
31. Knappe V, Frank F, Rohde E. Principles of lasers and biophotonic effects. Photomed Laser Surg 2004;22(5):411–7.
32. Ben Hatit Y, Blum R, Severin C, et al. The effects of the pulsed Nd:YAG laser on subgingival bacterial flora and on cementum. An in vivo study. J Clin Laser Med Surg 1996;14(3):137–43.
33. Radvar M, MacFarlane TW, MacKenzie D, et al. An evaluation of the Nd:YAG laser in periodontal pocket therapy. Br Dent J 1996;180(2):57–62.
34. Neill ME, Mellonig JT. Clinical effects of the Nd:YAG laser for combination periodontitis therapy. Pract Periodont Aesthetic Dent 1997;9(Suppl 6):1–5.
35. Liu CM, Hou LT, Wong MY, et al. Comparison of Nd:YAG laser versus scaling and root planing in periodontal therapy. J Periodontol 1999;70(11):1276–82.
36. Gutknecht N, Radufi P, Franzen R, et al. Reduction of specific microorganisms in periodontal pockets with the aid of an Nd:YAG laser – an in vivo study. J Oral Laser Appl 2002;2(3):175–80.
37. Sjostrom L, Friskopp J. Laser treatment as an adjunct to debridement of periodontal pockets. Swed Dent J 2002;26(2):51–7.
38. Miyazaki A, Yamaguchi T, Nishikata J, et al. Effects of Nd:YAG and CO_2 laser treatment and ultrasonic scaling on periodontal pockets of chronic periodontitis patients. J Periodontol 2003;74(2):175–80.
39. Harris DM, Gregg RH, McCarthy DK, et al. Laser-assisted new attachment procedure in private practice. Gen Dent 2004;52(5):386–403.

40. Noguchi T, Sanaoka A, Fukuda M, et al. Combined effects of Nd:YAG laser irradiation with local antibiotic applications into periodontal pockets. J Int Acad Periodontol 2005;7(1):8–15.
41. Verhagen LAM, Ellis JL. Comparison of adjunctive Nd:YAG laser treatment to anti-microbial treatment. J Oral Laser Appl 2006;6(2):29–37.
42. Beaumont RH, O'Leary TJ, Kafrawy AH. Relative resistance of long junctional epithelium adhesions and connective tissue attachments to plaque induced inflammation. J Periodontol 1984;55(4):213–23.
43. Magnuson I, Runstad L, Nyman S, et al. A long junctional epithelium – a locus, minoris resistentiae in plaque infection? J Clin Periodontol 1983;10(3):333–40.
44. Schwarz F, Sculean A, Georg T, et al. Clinical evaluation of the Er:YAG laser in combination with an enamel matrix protein derivative for the treatment of intrab-ony periodontal defects: a pilot study. J Clin Periodontol 2003;30(11):975–81.
45. Sculean A, Schwarz F, Berakdar M, et al. Healing of intrabony defects with or without an Er:YAG Laser. J Clin Periodontol 2004;31(8):604–8.
46. Yukna RA, Carr RL, Evans GH. Histologic evaluation of an Nd:YAG laser-assisted new attachment procedure in humans. Int J Periodontics Restorative Dent 2007; 27(6):577–87.
47. Magnusson I, Clark WB, Marks RG, et al. Attachment level measurements with a constant force electronic probe. J Clin Periodontol 1988;15(3):185–8.
48. Gibbs CH, Hirschfeld JW, Lee JG, et al. Description and clinical evaluation of a new computerized periodontal probe–the Florida probe. J Clin Periodontol 1988;15(2):137–44.
49. Schwarz F, Jeppsen S, Herten M, et al. A immunohistochemical characteriza-tion of periodontal wound healing following non-surgical treatment with fluores-cence controlled Er:YAG laser radiation in dogs. Lasers Surg Med 2007;39(5): 428–40.
50. Paster BJ, Olsen I, Aas JA, et al. The breadth of bacterial diversity in the human periodontal pocket and other oral sites. Periodontol 2000 2006;42:80–7.
51. Aoki A, Sasaki K, Watanabe H, et al. Lasers in non-surgical periodontal therapy. Periodontol 2000 2004;36:59–97.
52. Ishikawa I, Aoki A, Takasaki A. Potential applications of erbium:YAG laser in periodontics. J Periodont Res 2004;39(4):275–85.
53. Aoki A, Miura M, Akiyama F, et al. In vitro evaluation of Er:YAG laser scaling of subgingival calculus in comparison with ultrasonic scaling. J Periodont Res 2000;35(5):266–77.
54. Frenzen M, Braun A, Aniol D. Er:YAG scaling of diseased root surfaces. J Periodontol 2002;73(5):524–30.
55. Crespi R, Romanos GE, Barone A, et al. Effect of Er:YAG laser on diseased root surfaces: an in vivo study. J Periodontol 2005;76(5):686–90.
56. Ando Y, Watanabe H, Ishikawa I. Bactericidal effect of erbium:YAG laser on periodontopathic bacteria. Lasers Surg Med 1996;19(2):190–200.
57. Yamaguchi H, Kobayashi K, Osada R, et al. Effects of irradiation on an erbium:YAG laser on root surfaces. J Periodontol 1997;68(12):1151–5.
58. Sasaki KM, Aoki A, Masuno H, et al. Compositional analysis of root cementum and dentin after Er:YAG laser irradiation compared with CO_2 lased and intact roots using Fourier transformed infrared spectroscopy. J Periodont Res 2002; 37(1):50–9.
59. Schwarz F, Sculean A, Georg T, et al. Periodontal treatment with an Er:YAG laser compared to scaling and root planing. A controlled clinical study. J Periodontol 2001;72(4):361–7.

60. Schwarz F, Sculean A, Berakdar M, et al. Clinical evaluation of an Er:YAG laser combined with scaling and root planing for nonsurgical periodontal treatment. A controlled, prospective clinical study. J Clin Periodontol 2003; 30(1):26–34.
61. Schwarz F, Sculean A, Berakdar M, et al. Periodontal treatment with an Er:YAG laser or scaling and root planing. A 2-year follow-up split-mouth study. J Periodontol 2003;74(5):590–6.
62. Sculean A, Schwarz F, Berakdar M, et al. Periodontal treatment with an Er:YAG laser compared to ultrasonic instrumentation: a pilot study. J Periodontol 2004; 75(7):966–73.
63. Tomasi C, Schander K, Dahlén G, et al. Short-term clinical and microbiologic effects of pocket debridement with an Er:YAG laser during periodontal maintenance. J Periodontol 2006;77(1):111–8.
64. Crespi R, Capparè P, Toscanelli I, et al. Effects of Er:YAG laser compared to ultrasonic scaler in periodontal treatment: a 2-year follow-up split-mouth clinical study. J Periodontol 2007;78(7):1195–200.
65. Gaspirc B, Skaleric U. Clinical evaluation of periodontal surgical treatment with an Er:YAG laser: 5-year results. J Periodontol 2007;78(10):1864–71.
66. Kelbauskiene S, Maciulskiene V. A pilot study of Er, Cr:YSGG laser therapy used as an adjunct to scaling and root planing in patients with early and moderate periodontitis. Stomatologija 2007;9(1):21–6.
67. Lopes BMV, Marcantonio RAC, Thompson GMA, et al. Short-term clinical and immunologic effects of scaling and root planing with Er:YAG laser in chronic periodontitis. J Periodontol 2008;79(7):1158–67.
68. Moritz A, Schoop U, Goharkhay K, et al. Treatment of periodontal pockets with a diode laser. Lasers Surg Med 1998;22(5):302–11.
69. Borrajo JL, Varela LG, Castro GL, et al. Diode laser (980 nm) as adjunct to scaling and root planing. Photomed Laser Surg 2004;22(6):509–12.
70. Qadri T, Miranda L, Tuner J, et al. The short-term effects of low-level lasers as adjunct therapy in the treatment of periodontal inflammation. J Clin Periodontol 2005;32(7):714–9.
71. Kreisler M, Al Haj H, d'Hoedt B. Clinical efficacy of semiconductor laser application as an adjunct to conventional scaling and root planing. Lasers Surg Med 2005;37(5):350–5.
72. Kamma JJ, Vasdekis VGS, Romanos GE. The short-term effect of diode laser (980 nm) treatment of aggressive periodontitis. Evaluation of clinical and microbiological parameters. J Oral Laser Appl 2006;6(2):111–21.
73. Romanos G, Nentwig GH. Diode laser (980 nm) in oral and maxillofacial surgical procedures: clinical observations based on clinical applications. J Clin laser Med Surg 1999;17(5):193–7.
74. Kreisler M, Meyer C, Stender E, et al. Effect of diode laser irradiation on attachment rate of periodontal ligament cells: an in vitro study. J Periodontol 2001; 72(10):1312–7.
75. Schwarz F, Sculean A, Berakdar M, et al. In vivo and in vitro effects of an Er:YAG laser, a GaAlAs diode laser and scaling and root planing on periodontally diseased root surfaces. A comparative histologic study. Lasers Surg Med 2003;32(5):359–66.
76. Sharman WM, Allen CM, van Lier JE. Photodynamic therapeutics: basic principles and clinical applications. Drug Discov Today 1999;4(11):507–17.
77. Dougherty TJ, Gomer CJ, Henderson BW, et al. Photodynamic therapy. J Natl Cancer Inst 1998;90(12):889–905.

78. Ochsner M. Photophysical and photobiological processes in the photodynamic therapy of tumors. J Photochem Photobiol B Biol 1997;39(1):1–18.
79. Moan J, Berg K. The photodegradation of porphyrins in cells that can be used to estimate the lifetime of singlet oxygen. Photochem Photobiol 1991;53(4):549–53.
80. Yilmaz S, Kuru B, Kuru L, et al. Effect of gallium arsenide diode laser on human periodontal disease: a microbiological and clinical study. Lasers Surg Med 2002; 30(1):60–6.
81. Andersen R, Loebel N, Hammond D, et al. Treatment of periodontal disease by photodisinfection compared to scaling and root planing. J Clin Dent 2007; 18(2):34–8.
82. de Oliveira RR, Schwartz-Filho HO, Novaes AB Jr, et al. Antimicrobial photodynamic therapy in the non-surgical treatment of aggressive periodontitis: a preliminary randomized controlled clinical study. J Periodontol 2007;78(6):965–73.
83. Braun A, Dehn C, Krause F, et al. Short-term clinical effects of adjunctive antimicrobial photodynamic therapy in periodontal treatment: a randomized clinical trial. J Clin Periodontol 2008;35(10):877–84.
84. de Oliveira RR, Schwartz-Filho HO, Novaes AB Jr, et al. Antimicrobial photodynamic therapy in the non-surgical treatment of aggressive periodontitis: cytokine profile in gingival crevicular fluid, preliminary results. J Periodontol 2009;80(1): 98–105.
85. Polansky R, Haas M, Heschl A, et al. Clinical effectiveness of photodynamic therapy in the treatment of periodontitis. J Clin Periodontol 2009;36(7):575–80.
86. Choi KH, Im SU, Kim CS, et al. Effect of the carbon dioxide laser on the clinical parameters and crevicular IL-1beta when used as an adjunct to gingival flap surgery. J Int Acad Periodontol 2004;6(1):29–36.

Regeneration of Periodontal Tissue: Bone Replacement Grafts

Mark A. Reynolds, DDS, PhD*,
Mary Elizabeth Aichelmann-Reidy, DDS,
Grishondra L. Branch-Mays, DDS, MS

KEYWORDS
- Bone grafts • Periodontal • Intrabony • Scaffold
- Regeneration • Bone substitutes

Bone replacement grafts are widely used to promote bone formation and periodontal regeneration. Conventional surgical approaches, such as open flap debridement, provide critical access to evaluate and detoxify root surfaces as well as establish improved periodontal form and architecture; however, these surgical techniques offer only limited potential in restoring or reconstituting component periodontal tissues. Bone grafting materials function, in part, as structural scaffolds and matrices for attachment and proliferation of anchorage-dependent osteoblasts (**Fig. 1**). A wide range of bone grafting materials, including bone grafts and bone graft substitutes, have been applied and evaluated clinically, including autografts, allografts, xenografts, and alloplasts (synthetic/semisynthetic materials). Although not all bone grafting materials support the formation of a new periodontal attachment apparatus, there is conclusive evidence that periodontal regeneration is achievable with bone replacement grafts in humans.[1]

The purpose of this review is to provide an overview of the biologic function and clinical application of bone replacement grafts for periodontal regeneration. Emphasis is placed on the clinical and biologic goals of periodontal regeneration as well as evidence-based treatment outcomes.

PERIODONTAL REGENERATION: CLINICAL AND BIOLOGIC GOALS

The biologic goal of periodontal regeneration is restoration of the periodontium to its original form and function. Periodontal *repair* is healing of the periodontium by tissue

Department of Periodontics, Dental School, University of Maryland, 650 West Baltimore Street, Baltimore, MD 21201, USA
* Corresponding author.
E-mail address: mreynolds@umaryland.edu (M.A. Reynolds).

Dent Clin N Am 54 (2010) 55–71
doi:10.1016/j.cden.2009.09.003
0011-8532/09/$ – see front matter © 2010 Elsevier Inc. All rights reserved.

dental.theclinics.com

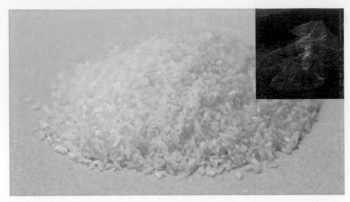

Fig. 1. Particulate bone grafts function, in part, by providing an osteoconductive matrix and structural framework for new bone formation. Demineralized bone matrix (DBM) also exhibits osteoinductivity. Particulate DBM (260–750 μm) is shown. Electron micrograph (*inset*) shows complex surface topography of a graft particle (×3000).

that does not fully restore the original functional anatomic and morphologic architecture. Following conventional surgical approaches, such as open flap debridement, repair of lost periodontal attachment occurs primarily through formation of a long junctional epithelium between the gingival flap and the previously diseased root surface. Epithelium is an efficient tissue for rapid wound repair, in part due to the comparatively high proliferation rate and effective adhesive mechanisms of epithelial cells.[2,3] Regenerative therapy, in contrast, is designed to support *regeneration* of the attachment apparatus, namely the formation of bone, cementum, and periodontal ligament (**Fig. 2**). Clinical outcome parameters consistent with successful regenerative therapy include reduced probing depth, increased clinical attachment level, and radiographic evidence of bone fill. At present, conclusive evidence of periodontal regeneration can be provided only through histologic evaluation of treated intraosseous defects using unambiguous reference points along the root surface (see **Fig. 2**).

BONE REPLACEMENT GRAFTS

Bone replacement grafts (bone grafts and bone graft substitutes) provide a structural framework for clot development, maturation, and remodeling that supports bone formation in osseous defects. Bone grafting materials also exhibit a variable capacity to promote the coordinated formation of bone, cementum, and periodontal ligament when placed and retained in periodontal defects. Bone grafting materials must possess the attributes of biocompatibility (lacking an immunogenic response) and osteoconductivity (providing a structure and surface topography that permit cellular attachment, proliferation, and migration). Bone replacement grafts may also possess other properties that support osteogenesis. *Osteogenic* grafting materials, such as cancellous bone/bone marrow, contain living cells that are capable of differentiation and formation of bone. *Osteoinductive* grafting materials, such as demineralized bone matrix (DBM), provide a biologic stimulus (proteins and growth factors) that induces the progression of mesenchymal stem cells and other osteoprogenitor cells toward the osteoblast lineage.

The Food and Drug Administration (FDA) regulates bone grafting materials that are intended to fill, augment, or reconstruct periodontal or bony defects of the oral and maxillofacial region. The regulatory control of the FDA includes human cells, tissues,

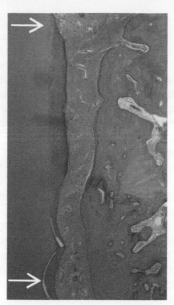

Fig. 2. Histologic evidence of periodontal regeneration (new bone, cementum, and periodontal ligament) following bone grafting with DBM. Note the reference notches (reference points for histologic measure of regenerated tissues) placed in the root to mark the pretreatment apical extent of calculus (*bottom arrow*) and height of the alveolar crest (*top arrow*) (H&E, original magnification ×25). (*Courtesy of* Dr Gerald M. Bowers, Pasadena, MD.)

and cellular-based products, under statutes published in Code of Federal Regulations (Federal Register, Title 21) that are intended for transplantation. Multiple classification systems have been used to organize bone replacement grafts, which commonly include source (eg, allograft), chemical composition (eg, calcium phosphate), and physical properties (eg, ceramic). Advances in material sciences, however, have increasingly blurred such boundaries between types of bone replacement grafts. For the purposes of this review, bone replacement grafts have been organized primarily according to source.

Autografts

The "gold standard" for bone grafting procedures historically has been particulate cancellous bone/bone marrow autografts, which can provide a rich source of bone and marrow cells that have osteogenic potential. Histologic findings from case reports substantiate the potential for autogenous bone/bone marrow grafts to support periodontal regeneration in humans.[4,5] Multiple clinical considerations have limited the use of extraoral autografts, particularly from iliac crest, including the possibility of surgical complications and pain associated with donor site.

Autogenous bone is frequently harvested from intraoral sites, often from the same quadrant as the regenerative surgery. Intraoral donor sites, however, typically yield comparatively limited graft volume. Harvesting sufficient donor bone, therefore, as an osseous coagulum of cortical or cortical-cancellous bone, can necessitate the creation of additional intraoral surgical sites, thereby increasing the potential for surgical morbidity and discomfort.

Allografts

Bone allograft is the most frequently used alternative to autogenous bone for bone grafting procedures in the United States. Under FDA regulations, facilities engaged in procuring and processing human tissues for transplantation must ensure that specified minimum medical screening and infectious disease testing have been performed, and that records exist and are maintained to document screening and testing for each human tissue. The American Association of Tissue Banks also sets standards, inspects facilities, and accredits tissue banks in North America. There are no reports of disease transmission during the 30-year history of use of freeze-dried bone allografts in periodontal therapy.[6]

Tissue banks process bone allografts using a variety of methods, some based on proprietary techniques, but most are based on similar underlying concepts that address cleansing, decontamination, antimicrobial treatment, dehydration, graft size, and terminal sterilization.[7] Particulate bone allografts are provided as mineralized or demineralized products. Allogeneic bone that has undergone extensive demineralization is referred to as DBM or demineralized freeze-dried bone allograft (DFDBA). DBM exhibits the capacity to induce bone formation in nonorthotopic sites, such as muscle, and is considered to be osteoinductive. Bone demineralized to levels of approximately 2% residual calcium has been shown to provide maximum osteoinductive potential by assay systems,[8] presumably due to exposure of bone morphogenetic proteins.[9] Bowers and colleagues[10,11] have provided conclusive histologic evidence that DBM supports periodontal regeneration in humans.

Xenografts

Xenografts are surgical grafts transplanted between different species. Two sources of xenografts are commercially marketed as particulate bone replacement grafts in clinical practice: bovine bone and natural coral. Anorganic bovine bone graft (ABM) is a naturally derived porous and deproteinized bovine bone mineral with comparable mineral composition and microporous structure to native humane bone.[12–15] ABM has been shown to support significant gains in clinical attachment level and hard tissue fill in human intrabony defects.[16] Available human histologic evidence provides proof-of-principle evidence that ABM[17] and ABM/collagen[18] can support periodontal regeneration in intrabony defects.

The calcium carbonate exoskeleton of coral species, such as Porites, can be converted to hydroxyapatite by hydrothermal exchange. Calcium carbonate-hydroxyapatite constructs can be produced by limited hydrothermal conversion.[19] The porosity and pore size distribution of hydroxyapatite, which is dependent primarily on coral species, provides a osteoconductive scaffold that enhances bone formation[20] and undergoes dissolution and resorption with bone remodeling.[21,22] Ripamonti and colleagues[19,23–26] have shown that coral-derived biomimetic matrices of different chemical compositions have the capacity to induce heterotopic bone formation in the nonhuman primate Papio ursinus.

Alloplasts

An alloplast is a biocompatible, inorganic synthetic bone grafting material. At present, alloplasts marketed for periodontal regeneration fall into 2 broad classes: ceramics and polymers. The composition, morphology, and surface topography of alloplasts provide the osteoconductive platform for promoting bone formation along the surface of the grafting material.[27] The fate of an alloplastic bone grafting material is dependent primarily on its chemical composition, structure, and physical properties.

Ceramic-based bone grafting materials have been widely used for bone and periodontal regeneration, and function primarily through osteoconduction. Commercially available ceramic-based materials include calcium phosphates (eg, tricalcium phosphate and hydroxyapatite), calcium sulfate, and bioactive glass. These ceramics have also been considered osteointegrative,[27] because of the tenacious, intimate bond formed between the new mineralized tissue and graft material.[28] Ceramics can exist in fully amorphous or crystalline phases, with the same ratios of elemental substances (calcium and phosphorus). Differences in the degree of crystalline arrangement significantly impact the physical and biologic characteristics of the ceramic, including strength, modulus, and dissolution rate.[29]

Synthetic and coral-derived porous hydroxyapatite has been shown to support significant clinical improvements in periodontal measures following implantation in intrabony defects.[1] The porosity and degree of sintering of synthetic hydroxyapatite ceramics primarily determines the rate of biodegradation—crystalline, nonporous hydroxyapatite is essentially nondegradable.[30] Human histologic evidence of ossification of the graft pores and the graft periphery of porous hydroxyapatite has been found in periodontal intrabony sites, with residual graft particles present 12 months following implantation.[31] Porous hydroxyapatite appears to exhibit osteoconductive properties, as reflected clinically in bone formation; however, no evidence of periodontal regeneration has been shown.

β-Tricalcium phosphate (β-TCP) is a porous form of calcium phosphate, with similar proportions of calcium and phosphate to cancellous bone.[32] As a bone grafting material, β-TCP supports improvements in clinical outcomes, including clinical attachment level, but histologic evidence reveals periodontal repair, primarily through the formation of a long junctional epithelial attachment, with limited new connective tissue attachment.[33–35] Although the surface layer of β-TCP allows for bone deposition in orthopedic sites,[28] including maxillary sinus augmentation,[36] this ceramic has been shown to become fibroencapsulated when placed in periodontal intrabony defects, failing to stimulate new bone growth, with residual graft particles evident 18 months following treatment.[33–35] Differences in the stoichiometric chemistry and structure of β-TCP may affect the rate of resorption and replacement with bone during healing.[36]

Bioactive glass is a ceramic composed principally of SiO_2. The original composition of bioactive glass approved by the FDA, designated 45S5, was composed of 46.1 mol% SiO_2, 26.9 mol% CaO, 24.4 mol% Na_2O, and 2.5 mol% P_2O_5.[37] The original composition and fine structure has been extensively modified in an attempt to further enhance bioactive glass as a bone replacement graft. Bioglass can bond directly to bone through the development of a surface layer of carbonated hydroxyapatite in situ.[37] This calcium phosphate-rich layer is thought to promote adsorption and concentration of osteoblast-derived proteins necessary for the mineralization of extracellular matrix.[38] Bioactive glass has been shown to significantly increase clinical attachment level and hard tissue fill when implanted in intrabony defects.[1] Although bioactive glass exhibits osteconductive properties as a grafting material in maxillary sinus[39,40] and extraction socket,[41–43] histologic analysis of human periodontal defects has revealed healing primarily by connective tissue encapsulation of the graft material and epithelial down-growth, with minimal evidence of new cementum or connective tissue attachment limited to the most apical part of the defect.[44,45]

Polymers can be classified based on source: natural and synthetic. Natural polymers that have been used in the fabrication of bone grafting materials include polysaccharides (eg, agarose, alginate, hyaluronic acid, chitosan) and polypeptides (eg, collagen, gelatin); however, the structural properties of natural polymers, including a comparatively weak mechanical strength and variable rates of degradation,[46] have limited their use as standalone bone grafting materials. Natural polymers may serve an important role in composite grafts, which incorporate a particulate or biologic, such as Bio-Oss Collagen (Geistlich Pharma AG, Wolhusen, Switzlerland).

Synthetic polymers (eg, poly(glycolic acid), poly(L-lactic acid), polyorthoester, polyanhydride) provide a platform for controlling the biomechanical properties of scaffolds as well as targeting drug delivery in tissue engineering.[47] Polymers are more widely used as barrier materials in guided tissue regeneration (GTR) procedures for the treatment of periodontal defects. At present, several polymer systems are being used for bone and periodontal regeneration, including polylactic acid (PLA)-based polymers and copolymers. These polymers have proved to be effective in periodontal applications as barrier materials[48] but can elicit inflammatory and foreign body reactions, especially following fragmentation secondary to bulk degradation.[49,50] Synthetic polymers have an expanded use in orthopedic applications as injectable and solid resin-based products.[27]

At present, a biocompatible microporous polymer containing polymethylmethacrylate (PMMA), polyhydroxylethylmethacrylate (PHEMA), and calcium hydroxide is available as a bone grafting material for the treatment of periodontal defects. This composite is prepared from a core of PMMA and PHEMA with a coating of calcium hydroxide. The polymer is hydrophilic and osteophilic, which purportedly aids in stabilization of the healing clot. A controlled study[51] and case series reports[52–55] provide evidence for the effectiveness of this polymeric grafting material in improving clinical parameters, relative to open flap debridement, in the treatment of periodontal intraosseous defects.[51] Histologic evaluations revealed that the polymer was associated with minimal inflammation and infrequent foreign body giant cells, with evidence of both bone apposition and soft tissue encapsulation, at 1 to 30 months following implantation.[51,55–57]

COMPOSITE GRAFTS

In periodontal regenerative procedures, bone replacement grafts have been widely used to expand the volume of autogenous bone for regenerative procedures when sufficient autogenous bone is not readily available. The bone replacement graft, therefore, serves as a graft expander or extender. In other regenerative applications, such as ridge and sinus augmentation whereby structural support is often necessary, the physical properties of the graft expander can be an important factor in regenerative outcome. Anorganic bovine graft material, for example, provides a stable osteoconductive structural framework or matrix for bone in-growth and undergoes minimal degradation and remodeling over comparatively long periods.[58–60] Recent advances in material sciences now permit the fabrication of polymeric and ceramic composite grafts, with biologic and physical properties optimized for specific tissue engineering applications.[61]

Strategies to improve the delivery and containment of bone replacement grafts have focused on agents that function as a graft carriers or binders. Human histologic evidence has shown that the presence of residual DBM particles is closely associated with the extent of periodontal regeneration.[62] Most carriers are solid gels or pastes, which are designed to resorb within several days of implantation. Carrier materials used in commercially marketed DBM-based products include Poloxamer 407, lecithin, hyaluronic acid, glycerol, porcine gelatin, and calcium sulfate, among others.[63] These carrier materials impart different properties to the particulate bone grafting material. Poloxamer 407, for example, is a reverse-phase polymer that is fluid at room temperature and becomes a firm gel at body temperature. In orthopedic applications, carrier materials have been implicated in differences in the efficacy[64] and potential safety of DBM products.[65,66]

BIOMIMETICS AND BIOLOGICS

Osteoblasts are anchorage-dependent cells that are highly responsive to the surface characteristics of osteoconductive scaffolds. Efforts to enhance the effectiveness of graft materials have focused on the use of biomimetic engineering and biologic agents, such as growth factors. PepGen P-15 (Dentsply Friadent, Mannheim, Germany) is bovine-derived hydroxyapatite (anorganic bone) that contains a short polypeptide chain of 15 amino acids, which is a biomimetic cell-binding region of type I collagen. The amino acid peptide, therefore, mimics type I collagen, the major component of bone matrix, promoting cell attachment, which may enhance osteogenesis. In vitro studies have shown that ABM carrying the cell-binding peptide P-15 promotes anchorage-dependent cell survival.[12] The efficacy of PepGen P-15 for the treatment of intrabony defects has been established in controlled clinical trials.[67,68]

The potential for growth factors to modify and enhance the regenerative capacity of bone grafts was highlighted in early studies examining the osteoinductive properties of DBM. Recent attention has focused on the potential for biologic mediators to improve wound healing and enhance the clinical benefits of bone replacement grafts. Platelet-rich plasma (PRP), collected by centrifugation of autogenous serum, provides a source of highly concentrated platelets, which produce growth factors that are critical for normal healing. When admixed with a bone graft, PRP facilitates graft placement and containment (**Fig. 3**). PRP has been shown to provide beneficial effects, as reflected in gains in clinical attachment level, when used as an adjunct to periodontal regenerative therapy.[69]

In 2005, the FDA approved for marketing a new dental bone filling device, GEM 21S (Osteohealth/Luitpold Pharmaceuticals, Inc, Shirley, NY), which combines recombinant human platelet-derived growth factor-BB (rhPDGF-BB) and β-TCP for the treatment of periodontal-related defects. GEM 21S is a completely synthetic grafting system and is the first dental bone grafting material with a recombinant growth factor approved by the FDA. GEM 21S contains over 1000 times the concentration of platelet-derived growth factor obtainable in current PRP preparations from the patient's own peripheral venous blood. PDGF-BB promotes angiogenesis as well as enhances cell recruitment and proliferation of bone and periodontal ligament cells.[70,71]

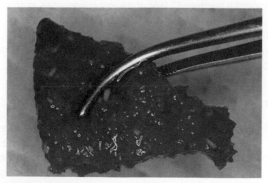

Fig. 3. Platelet-rich plasma provides a source of autogenous growth factors and can facilitate graft placement and containment. (*Courtesy of* Dr James D. Kassolis, Baltimore, MD.)

The efficacy and safety of GEM 21S for the treatment of intrabony defects has been established in a large-scale multicenter, randomized controlled clinical trial.[72]

BONE GRAFT THERAPY
Surgery

Bone graft therapy builds on the basic principles of periodontal surgical technique, including appropriate case selection and preoperative management. Complete defect debridement and root surface decontamination are essential before placement of the bone graft material. The most notable difference in surgical technique involves gingival flap design, because primary and passive flap closure are critical for ensuring wound closure. In general, full-thickness mucoperiosteal flaps are elevated using sulcular incisions to conserve the papillary and keratinized tissue, ensuring the flap can be adapted at a more coronal level postoperatively. This procedure will aid the development of space for the graft material and stability of the healing clot at a more coronal level than the prior diseased attachment level. The flap design, when possible, ideally avoids placing an incision directly over the defect site, because the defect site does not provide direct periosteal blood supply and lacks optimal structural support of the incision margins. Following thorough root debridement and preparation of the defect site under magnification and supplemental illumination, the bone grafting material is implanted into the defect, lightly condensed, and contoured to mimic the normal architecture of adjacent alveolar process. The mucoperiosteal flaps are mobilized to permit tension-free coaptation and primary closure with sutures (**Fig. 4**). The most commonly reported untoward event following bone graft therapy in controlled clinical trials has been partial loss (exfoliation) of graft particles postoperatively.[1] Evidence of retained or residual DBM graft particles has been shown to be closely associated with the extent of periodontal regeneration in histologic analysis.[62]

Root Surface Biomodification

The topical application of chemical agents to modify the root surface is among one of the earliest reported clinical approaches to prepare root surfaces for optimal attachment of periodontal tissues and regeneration.[73] Several agents, such as citric acid, tetracycline, and ethylenediamine tetra-acetic acid (EDTA), have been shown to result in surface biomodification, including detoxification, demineralization, and collagen fiber exposure. A recent systematic review, however, concluded that chemical root modifiers do not enhance reductions in probing depth or gains in clinical attachment level following periodontal surgery.[74] Because improvements in clinical measures can occur following periodontal repair—via a long junctional epithelium, connective tissue attachment, or both—as well as periodontal regeneration, many clinicians continue to routinely apply root modifiers in an effort to promote true regeneration, namely the formation of new bone, cementum, and periodontal ligament.

PERIODONTAL DEFECTS AND REGENERATIVE SUCCESS

Periodontitis results in destructive changes in the component hard and soft tissues of the periodontium, culminating in loss of supporting alveolar bone and periodontal attachment. Horizontal patterns of alveolar bone loss are not amenable to periodontal regeneration with current regenerative therapies, including bone grafts. Vertical or angular bony defects, including furcation defects, are often responsive to periodontal regeneration.

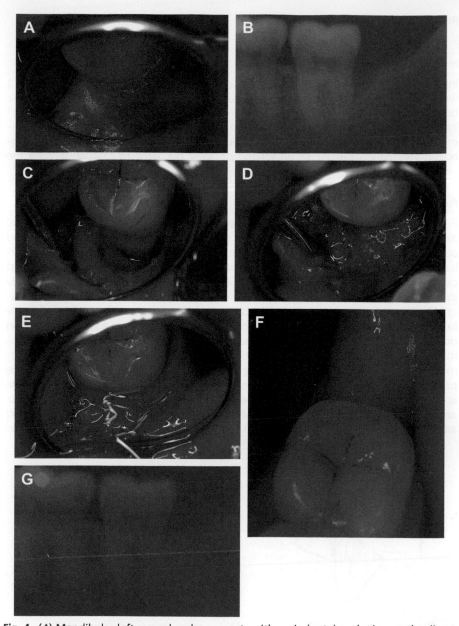

Fig. 4. (*A*) Mandibular left second molar presents with periodontal pocketing on the direct distal. Patient is a nonsmoker and demonstrates excellent oral hygiene. (*Courtesy of* Dr Paul S. Rosen, Yardley, PA.) (*B*) Preoperative radiograph reveals evidence of an advanced intrabony defect on the distal aspect of the tooth. (*C*) Elevation of facial and lingual flaps using sulcular incisions, preserving the papilla, exposes a 3-wall intrabony defect measuring 6 mm from base to the alveolar crest on the distal of the second molar. Rotary instrumentation using a multifluted surgical length burr was used to plane the root surface to the depth of the defect. Small perforations are made to decorticate the bony walls of the defect, followed by the topical application of citric acid (pH 1.0) to decontaminate and condition the root surface. (*D*) Mineralized freeze-dried bone allograft admixed with calcium sulfate is placed with light incremental pressure until the bone graft slightly overfills of the defect. (*E*) Primary closure of the flaps is achieved using expanded polytetrafluoroethylene sutures (Gore-Tex; W.L. Gore and Associates, Inc, Newark, DE). (*F*) Clinical presentation of the surgical site 1 year following bone grafting surgery. (*G*) Postoperative radiograph suggests remodeling of the graft with nearly complete resolution of the intrabony defect.

Intrabony Defects

Intrabony defects are commonly described by the number of bony walls (1, 2, or 3 walls) and depth of the defect (measured from the crestal height of bone to the base of the defect) (**Fig. 5**). Periodontal probing and transgingival bone "sounding" can provide important diagnostic information to aid the appropriate selection of regenerative therapy for intrabony defects.[75] Radiographs also provide important diagnostic information related to defect morphology but generally underestimate the severity of bone loss.[76]

Furcation Defects

Furcation invasion is most commonly classified according to the degree of horizontal extension within the furcation. The degree of furcation involvement is often classified as Class I (incipient loss of bone limited to the furcation flute that does not extend horizontally within the furcation), Class II (variable bone loss that does not extend completely through the furcation), and Class III (bone loss extending completely through the furcation).[77]

Although early or incipient Class I furcation defects are generally considered maintainable by nonsurgical therapy and effective plaque control, more advanced furcation defects (Class II and Class III) usually require surgical management for effective inflammatory disease control and tooth retention.[77] Surgery permits access for root debridement, detoxification, and odontoplasty to promote periodontal regeneration. The primary clinical objective in the regenerative treatment of Class II furcation defects is closure of the furcation entrance to the oral environment. Class III furcation defects are generally not amenable to successful regenerative therapy, and are usually treated with surgical debridement and apical positioning of the flap to obtain pocket

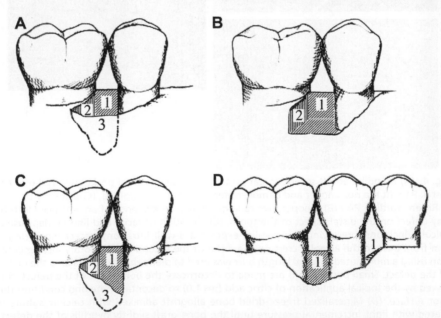

Fig. 5. Schematic illustration of intraosseous defects classified according to the number of bony walls present. (*A*) Three-wall defect; (*B*) 2-wall defect; (*C*) combination defect; (*D*) 1-wall defect. One-wall defects typically do not respond well to regenerative therapy.

reduction, thereby facilitating access for plaque control, or hemisection of the tooth to eliminate the furcation.

CASE SELECTION

In general, early or shallow intrabony lesions (defects of 3 mm or less) and Class I (incipient) furcation defects can be effectively managed using nonsurgical or nonregenerative surgical therapies. Early intrabony defects are thought to have less potential for regeneration due, in part, to a limited potential for space development for holding graft particles and concomitant crestal bone resorption during healing.[78] Given adequate surgical access, the most predictable regenerative outcomes are typically achieved in narrow 3-wall defects[79] as well as Class II furcation defects with proximal bone height at or above the level of the furcation entrance.[80]

TREATMENT OUTCOMES: EXPECTATIONS BASED ON EVIDENCE-BASED REVIEWS
Intrabony Defects

Systematic reviews of randomized controlled trials provide strong evidence that bone replacement grafts support improvements in clinical parameters, including probing depth, clinical attachment level, and defect fill, when compared with open flap debridement alone in intrabony defects (**Table 1**).[1,81–83] Literature-based estimates of bone fill range from 2.3 to 3.0 mm or 60% of the defect following grafting of intrabony defects.[84] Particulate bone grafting materials also seem to reduce crestal bone loss, whereas barrier materials may increase recession of the gingival margin.[1,48] When particulate graft is combined with a barrier, modest but nonsignificant improvement in bone levels is obtained, with significant attachment level gain and probing depth reduction when compared with graft alone.[1]

Comparisons in treatment outcomes, such as defect fill, obtained in different studies must be made with caution. Laurell and colleagues[78] reviewed all observational and controlled studies published during a 20-year period on the surgical treatment of intrabony defects with open flap debridement, GTR, and bone grafts. Defect

Table 1
Mean change in clinical measures following bone replacement graft therapy

Bone Replacement Graft	N	Clinical Attachment Level (mm)	N	Probing Depth (mm)	N	Defect Fill (mm)
Allograft	12	1.6 ± 1.3	10	2.9 ± 1.6	13	2.2 ± 1.4
Autograft	3	2.6 ± 1.2	1	1.4 ± 1.0	2	2.2 ± 1.2
Synthetic hydroxyapatite	4	2.8 ± 1.7	7	3.2 ± 1.4	6	2.1 ± 1.3
Coralline hydroxyapatite	4	2.3 ± 1.4	4	3.2 ± 1.5	3	2.8 ± 1.2
Bioactive glass	4	2.3 ± 1.8	4	3.4 ± 1.8	4	2.6 ± 1.0
PepGen P-15	1	1.3 ± 1.9	1	2.4 ± 1.5	1	2.8 ± 1.2
GEM 21S	1	3.7 ± 0.2	1	4.4 ± 0.2	1	2.5 ± 0.3[a]

Values represent mean ± standard deviation, where N = number of studies.
Summary statistics are derived from randomized controlled studies. *Reported in* Reynolds et al[1] (allograft, autograft, synthetic hydroxyapatite, coralline hydroxyapatite, bioactive glass); Yukna et al[67] (PepGen P-15); Nevins et al[93] (GEM 21S).
[a] Hard tissue measurements by radiographic assessment.

fill was found to be positively correlated with initial defect depth following open flap debridement and grafting procedures, as reported by others. Differences in mean defect fill parallel initial differences in average pretreatment defect depth, making direct quantitative comparisons of improvements (effect sizes) across studies difficult to evaluate and vulnerable to confounding.

Histologic evidence of periodontal regeneration in intraosseous defects has been reported most extensively for autogenous bone and DFDBA, although case reports provide proof-of-principle of regeneration for other bone grafting materials, such as PepGen P-15,[85] Bio-Oss Collagen (anorganic bovine-derived bone matrix and collagen),[86] and GEM 21S.[87] In contrast, open flap debridement and alloplastic grafts support primarily periodontal repair, which is characterized by formation of a long junctional epithelium.[1]

Furcation Defects

Systematic reviews provide strong evidence that Class II furcations respond most favorably and predictably to a combinatorial approach using GTR and a bone grafting material together.[48] Using this combination therapy, Bowers and colleagues[80] achieved the highest rate of complete furcation closure in mandibular molar Class II facial defects, with horizontal probing depths of 5 mm or less and interproximal bone at or above the level of the furcation entrance. In general, the more advanced the furcation defect, the less favorable the prognosis for complete periodontal regeneration and furcation closure. Early treatment of furcation defects, therefore, is critical for improving the overall prognosis.

FACTORS IMPACTING TREATMENT OUTCOME

The success of regenerative therapy is influenced by multiple factors related to the patient, periodontal defect, and surgical management,[88,89] which contribute to variability in clinical outcomes following regenerative therapy.[90] Defect morphology and root configuration can affect both surgical access and containment of the bone replacement graft, thereby influencing treatment outcome. Patient compliance with recommended oral hygiene procedures and supportive periodontal maintenance programs are essential for achieving an optimal regenerative outcome and long-term therapeutic success. Finally, smoking adversely affects wound healing, including periodontal regeneration, and increases the risk for periodontal breakdown following treatment.[91,92]

SUMMARY

Controlled clinical trials provide strong evidence for the effectiveness of bone replacement grafts in the treatment of periodontal defects. The potential for selected bone replacement grafts, such as DBM, to support true periodontal regeneration, including new bone, cementum, and periodontal ligament, has been well established through histologic analysis in humans. Most current bone grafting materials are osteoconductive and function as passive matrices for ingrowth of osteoprogenitor tissue. Composite grafting materials, incorporating biomimetic and biologic components, have shown great potential to enhance regenerative outcomes. Future bone grafting materials will likely build on innovative polymeric and ceramic platforms with controlled biophysical properties that enable the targeted delivery of drugs, biologics, and cells, thereby improving the degree and predictability of periodontal regeneration.

REFERENCES

1. Reynolds MA, Aichelmann-Reidy ME, Branch-Mays GL, et al. The efficacy of bone replacement grafts in the treatment of periodontal osseous defects. A systematic review. Ann Periodontol 2003;8:227.
2. Shimono M, Ishikawa T, Enokiya Y, et al. Biological characteristics of the junctional epithelium. J Electron Microsc (Tokyo) 2003;52:627.
3. Nievers MG, Schaapveld RQ, Sonnenberg A. Biology and function of hemidesmosomes. Matrix Biol 1999;18:5.
4. Hiatt WH, Schallhorn RG, Aaronian AJ. The induction of new bone and cementum formation. IV. Microscopic examination of the periodontium following human bone and marrow allograft, autograft and nongraft periodontal regenerative procedures. J Periodontol 1978;49:495.
5. Ross SE, Cohen DW. The fate of a free osseous tissue autograft. A clinical and histologic case report. Periodontics 1968;6:145.
6. Centers for Disease Control and Prevention: Bone allografts. What is the risk of disease transmission with bone allografts? In: Department of Health and Human Services. Available at: http://www.cd.gov/OralHealth/Infectioncontrol/faq/allografts.htm. Accessed September 30, 2009.
7. Holtzclaw D, Toscano N, Eisenlohr L, et al. The safety of bone allografts used in dentistry: a review. J Am Dent Assoc 2008;139:1192.
8. Zhang M, Powers RM Jr, Wolfinbarger L Jr. Effect(s) of the demineralization process on the osteoinductivity of demineralized bone matrix. J Periodontol 1997;68:1085.
9. Urist MR. Bone: formation by autoinduction. Science 1965;150:893.
10. Bowers G, Felton F, Middleton C, et al. Histologic comparison of regeneration in human intrabony defects when osteogenin is combined with demineralized freeze-dried bone allograft and with purified bovine collagen. J Periodontol 1991;62:690.
11. Bowers GM, Chadroff B, Carnevale R, et al. Histologic evaluation of new attachment apparatus formation in humans. Part III. J Periodontol 1989;60:683.
12. Hanks T, Atkinson BL. Comparison of cell viability on anorganic bone matrix with or without P-15 cell binding peptide. Biomaterials 2004;25:4831.
13. Rosen VB, Hobbs LW, Spector M. The ultrastructure of anorganic bovine bone and selected synthetic hyroxyapatites used as bone graft substitute materials. Biomaterials 2002;23:921.
14. Fulmer NL, Bussard GM, Gampper TJ, et al. Anorganic bovine bone and analogs of bone mineral as implants for craniofacial surgery: a literature review. J Long Term Eff Med Implants 1998;8:69.
15. Spector M. Anorganic bovine bone and ceramic analogs of bone mineral as implants to facilitate bone regeneration. Clin Plast Surg 1994;21:437.
16. Richardson CR, Mellonig JT, Brunsvold MA, et al. Clinical evaluation of Bio-Oss: a bovine-derived xenograft for the treatment of periodontal osseous defects in humans. J Clin Periodontol 1999;26:421.
17. Mellonig JT. Human histologic evaluation of a bovine-derived bone xenograft in the treatment of periodontal osseous defects. Int J Periodontics Restorative Dent 2000;20:19.
18. Nevins ML, Camelo M, Lynch SE, et al. Evaluation of periodontal regeneration following grafting intrabony defects with bio-oss collagen: a human histologic report. Int J Periodontics Restorative Dent 2003;23:9.
19. Ripamonti U, Crooks J, Khoali L, et al. The induction of bone formation by coral-derived calcium carbonate/hydroxyapatite constructs. Biomaterials 2009;30:1428.

20. Damien E, Revell PA. Coralline hydroxyapatite bone graft substitute: a review of experimental studies and biomedical applications. J Appl Biomat Biomech 2004;2:65.
21. Guillemin G, Meunier A, Dallant P, et al. Comparison of coral resorption and bone apposition with two natural corals of different porosities. J Biomed Mater Res 1989;23:765.
22. Guillemin G, Patat JL, Fournie J, et al. The use of coral as a bone graft substitute. J Biomed Mater Res 1987;21:557.
23. Ripamonti U. The morphogenesis of bone in replicas of porous hydroxyapatite obtained from conversion of calcium carbonate exoskeletons of coral. J Bone Joint Surg Am 1991;73:692.
24. Ripamonti U. Calvarial reconstruction in baboons with porous hydroxyapatite. J Craniofac Surg 1992;3:149.
25. Ripamonti U. Osteoinduction in porous hydroxyapatite implanted in heterotopic sites of different animal models. Biomaterials 1996;17:31.
26. Ripamonti U, Van den Heever B, Van Wyk J. Expression of the osteogenic phenotype in porous hydroxyapatite implanted extraskeletally in baboons. Matrix 1993; 13:491.
27. Laurencin C, Khan Y, El-Amin SF. Bone graft substitutes. Expert Rev Med Devices 2006;3:49.
28. Boccaccini AR, Blaker JJ. Bioactive composite materials for tissue engineering scaffolds. Expert Rev Med Devices 2005;2:303.
29. Lemons JE. Bioceramics. Is there a difference? Clin Orthop Relat Res 1990;261: 153.
30. Klein CP, Driessen AA, de Groot K, et al. Biodegradation behavior of various calcium phosphate materials in bone tissue. J Biomed Mater Res 1983;17:769.
31. Stahl SS, Froum SJ. Histologic and clinical responses to porous hydroxylapatite implants in human periodontal defects. Three to twelve months postimplantation. J Periodontol 1987;58:689.
32. Hashimoto-Uoshima M, Ishikawa I, Kinoshita A, et al. Clinical and histologic observation of replacement of biphasic calcium phosphate by bone tissue in monkeys. Int J Periodontics Restorative Dent 1995;15:205.
33. Baldock WT, Hutchens LH Jr, McFall WT Jr, et al. An evaluation of tricalcium phosphate implants in human periodontal osseous defects of two patients. J Periodontol 1985;56:1.
34. Stahl SS, Froum S. Histological evaluation of human intraosseous healing responses to the placement of tricalcium phosphate ceramic implants. I. Three to eight months. J Periodontol 1986;57:211.
35. Froum S, Stahl SS. Human intraosseous healing responses to the placement of tricalcium phosphate ceramic implants. II. 13 to 18 months. J Periodontol 1987; 58:103.
36. Chopra PM, Johnson M, Nagy TR, et al. Micro-computed tomographic analysis of bone healing subsequent to graft placement. J Biomed Mater Res B Appl Biomater 2009;88:611.
37. Hench LL, Paschall HA. Direct chemical bond of bioactive glass-ceramic materials to bone and muscle. J Biomed Mater Res 1973;7:25.
38. Schepers E, de Clercq M, Ducheyne P, et al. Bioactive glass particulate material as a filler for bone lesions. J Oral Rehabil 1991;18:439.
39. Galindo-Moreno P, Avila G, Fernandez-Barbero JE, et al. Clinical and histologic comparison of two different composite grafts for sinus augmentation: a pilot clinical trial. Clin Oral Implants Res 2008;19:755.

40. Scarano A, Degidi M, Iezzi G, et al. Maxillary sinus augmentation with different biomaterials: a comparative histologic and histomorphometric study in man. Implant Dent 2006;15:197.
41. Stvrtecky R, Gorustovich A, Perio C, et al. A histologic study of bone response to bioactive glass particles used before implant placement: a clinical report. J Prosthet Dent 2003;90:424.
42. Norton MR, Wilson J. Dental implants placed in extraction sites implanted with bioactive glass: human histology and clinical outcome. Int J Oral Maxillofac Implants 2002;17:249.
43. Froum S, Cho SC, Rosenberg E, et al. Histological comparison of healing extraction sockets implanted with bioactive glass or demineralized freeze-dried bone allograft: a pilot study. J Periodontol 2002;73:94.
44. Nevins ML, Camelo M, Nevins M, et al. Human histologic evaluation of bioactive ceramic in the treatment of periodontal osseous defects. Int J Periodontics Restorative Dent 2000;20:458.
45. Sculean A, Windisch P, Keglevich T, et al. Clinical and histologic evaluation of an enamel matrix protein derivative combined with a bioactive glass for the treatment of intrabony periodontal defects in humans. Int J Periodontics Restorative Dent 2005;25:139.
46. Lee K, Kaplan D, editors. Tissue engineering I. Scaffold systems for tissue engineering, Advances in biochemical engineering/biotechnology, vol. 102. New York: Springer; 2006.
47. Sokolsky-Papkov M, Agashi K, Olaye A, et al. Polymer carriers for drug delivery in tissue engineering. Adv Drug Deliv Rev 2007;59:187.
48. Murphy KG, Gunsolley JC. Guided tissue regeneration for the treatment of periodontal intrabony and furcation defects. A systematic review. Ann Periodontol 2003;8:266.
49. Polimeni G, Koo KT, Pringle GA, et al. Histopathological observations of a polylactic acid-based device intended for guided bone/tissue regeneration. Clin Implant Dent Relat Res 2008;10:99.
50. Danesh-Meyer MJ, Wikesjo UM. Gingival recession defects and guided tissue regeneration: a review. J Periodont Res 2001;36:341.
51. Yukna RA. HTR polymer grafts in human periodontal osseous defects. I. 6-month clinical results. J Periodontol 1990;61:633.
52. Calongne KB, Aichelmann-Reidy ME, Yukna RA, et al. Clinical comparison of microporous biocompatible composite of PMMA, PHEMA and calcium hydroxide grafts and expanded polytetrafluoroethylene barrier membranes in human mandibular molar Class II furcations. A case series. J Periodontol 2001;72:1451.
53. Haris AG, Szabo G, Ashman A, et al. Five-year 224-patient prospective histological study of clinical applications using a synthetic bone alloplast. Implant Dent 1998;7:287.
54. Yukna RA, Yukna CN. Six-year clinical evaluation of HTR synthetic bone grafts in human grade II molar furcations. J Periodont Res 1997;32:627.
55. Yukna RA, Greer RO Jr. Human gingival tissue response to HTR polymer. J Biomed Mater Res 1992;26:517.
56. Stahl SS, Froum SJ, Tarnow D. Human clinical and histologic responses to the placement of HTR polymer particles in 11 intrabony lesions. J Periodontol 1990;61:269.
57. Froum SJ. Human histologic evaluation of HTR polymer and freeze-dried bone allograft. A case report. J Clin Periodontol 1996;23:615.

58. Iezzi G, Scarano A, Mangano C, et al. Histologic results from a human implant retrieved due to fracture 5 years after insertion in a sinus augmented with anorganic bovine bone. J Periodontol 2008;79:192.
59. Traini T, Valentini P, Iezzi G, et al. A histologic and histomorphometric evaluation of anorganic bovine bone retrieved 9 years after a sinus augmentation procedure. J Periodontol 2007;78:955.
60. Sartori S, Silvestri M, Forni F, et al. Ten-year follow-up in a maxillary sinus augmentation using anorganic bovine bone (Bio-Oss). A case report with histomorphometric evaluation. Clin Oral Implants Res 2003;14:369.
61. Hutmacher DW, Schantz JT, Lam CX, et al. State of the art and future directions of scaffold-based bone engineering from a biomaterials perspective. J Tissue Eng Regen Med 2007;1:245.
62. Reynolds MA, Bowers GM. Fate of demineralized freeze-dried bone allografts in human intrabony defects. J Periodontol 1996;67:150.
63. Borden M. The development of bone graft materials using various formulations of demineralized bone matrix. In: Laurencin CT, editor. Bone graft substitutes. West Conshohocken (PA): ASTM International. 2003. Chapter 5. p. 96
64. Drosos GI, Kazakos KI, Kouzoumpasis P, et al. Safety and efficacy of commercially available demineralised bone matrix preparations: a critical review of clinical studies. Injury 2007;38(Suppl 4):S13.
65. Wang JC, Kanim LE, Nagakawa IS, et al. Dose-dependent toxicity of a commercially available demineralized bone matrix material. Spine (Phila Pa 1976) 2001; 26:1429.
66. Bostrom MP, Yang X, Kennan M, et al. An unexpected outcome during testing of commercially available demineralized bone graft materials: how safe are the nonallograft components? Spine (Phila Pa 1976) 2001;26:1425.
67. Yukna RA, Callan DP, Krauser JT, et al. Multi-center clinical evaluation of combination anorganic bovine-derived hydroxyapatite matrix (ABM)/cell binding peptide (P-15) as a bone replacement graft material in human periodontal osseous defects. 6-month results. J Periodontol 1998;69:655.
68. Yukna RA, Krauser JT, Callan DP, et al. Multi-center clinical comparison of combination anorganic bovine-derived hydroxyapatite matrix (ABM)/cell binding peptide (P-15) and ABM in human periodontal osseous defects. 6-month results. J Periodontol 2000;71:1671.
69. Plachokova AS, Nikolidakis D, Mulder J, et al. Effect of platelet-rich plasma on bone regeneration in dentistry: a systematic review. Clin Oral Implants Res 2008;19:539.
70. Hollinger JO, Hart CE, Hirsch SN, et al. Recombinant human platelet-derived growth factor: biology and clinical applications. J Bone Joint Surg Am 2008; 90(Suppl 1):48.
71. Oates TW, Rouse CA, Cochran DL. Mitogenic effects of growth factors on human periodontal ligament cells in vitro. J Periodontol 1993;64:142.
72. Nevins M, Camelo M, Nevins ML, et al. Periodontal regeneration in humans using recombinant human platelet-derived growth factor-BB (rhPDGF-BB) and allogenic bone. J Periodontol 2003;74:1282.
73. Lowenguth RA, Blieden TM. Periodontal regeneration: root surface demineralization. Periodontol 2000 1993;1:54.
74. Mariotti A. Efficacy of chemical root surface modifiers in the treatment of periodontal disease. A systematic review. Ann Periodontol 2003;8:205.
75. Kim HY, Yi SW, Choi SH, et al. Bone probing measurement as a reliable evaluation of the bone level in periodontal defects. J Periodontol 2000;71:729.

76. Eickholz P, Kim TS, Benn DK, et al. Validity of radiographic measurement of interproximal bone loss. Oral Surg Oral Med Oral Pathol Oral Radiol Endod 1998;85:99.

77. Carranza FA Jr, Jolkovsky DL. Current status of periodontal therapy for furcation involvements. Dent Clin North Am 1991;35:555.

78. Laurell L, Gottlow J, Zybutz M, et al. Treatment of intrabony defects by different surgical procedures. A literature review. J Periodontol 1998;69:303.

79. Cortellini P, Bowers GM. Periodontal regeneration of intrabony defects: an evidence-based treatment approach. Int J Periodontics Restorative Dent 1995; 15:128.

80. Bowers GM, Schallhorn RG, McClain PK, et al. Factors influencing the outcome of regenerative therapy in mandibular Class II furcations: part I. J Periodontol 2003; 74:1255.

81. Needleman I, Tucker R, Giedrys-Leeper E, et al. A systematic review of guided tissue regeneration for periodontal infrabony defects. J Periodontal Res 2002; 37:380.

82. Trombelli L, Heitz-Mayfield LJ, Needleman I, et al. A systematic review of graft materials and biological agents for periodontal intraosseous defects. J Clin Periodontol 2002;29(Suppl 3):117.

83. Trombelli L. Which reconstructive procedures are effective for treating the periodontal intraosseous defect? Periodontol 2000 2005;37:88.

84. Brunsvold MA, Mellonig JT. Bone grafts and periodontal regeneration. Periodontol 2000 1993;1:80.

85. Yukna R, Salinas TJ, Carr RF. Periodontal regeneration following use of ABM/P-1 5: a case report. Int J Periodontics Restorative Dent 2002;22:146.

86. Hartman GA, Arnold RM, Mills MP, et al. Clinical and histologic evaluation of anorganic bovine bone collagen with or without a collagen barrier. Int J Periodontics Restorative Dent 2004;24:127.

87. Ridgway HK, Mellonig JT, Cochran DL. Human histologic and clinical evaluation of recombinant human platelet-derived growth factor and beta-tricalcium phosphate for the treatment of periodontal intraosseous defects. Int J Periodontics Restorative Dent 2008;28:171.

88. Garrett S. Periodontal regeneration around natural teeth. Ann Periodontol 1996;1: 621.

89. Wang HL, Cooke J. Periodontal regeneration techniques for treatment of periodontal diseases. Dent Clin North Am 2005;49:637.

90. Aichelmann-Reidy ME, Reynolds MA. Predictability of clinical outcomes following regenerative therapy in intrabony defects. J Periodontol 2008;79:387.

91. Rosen PS, Marks MH, Reynolds MA. Influence of smoking on long-term clinical results of intrabony defects treated with regenerative therapy. J Periodontol 1996;67:1159.

92. Johnson GK, Hill M. Cigarette smoking and the periodontal patient. J Periodontol 2004;75:196.

93. Nevins M, Giannobile WV, McGuire MK, et al. Platelet-derived growth factor stimulates bone fill and rate of attachment level gain: results of a large multicenter randomized controlled trial. J Periodontol 2005;76:2205.

Regeneration of Periodontal Tissues: Guided Tissue Regeneration

Cristina C. Villar, DDS, MS, PhD*, David L. Cochran, DDS, MS, PhD, MMSc

KEYWORDS

• Guided tissue regeneration • Membranes • Intrabony defects
• Furcation defects • Periodontal regeneration

The ultimate goal of periodontal therapy is to prevent further attachment loss and predictably restore the periodontal supporting structures that were lost because of disease or trauma in a way that the architecture and function of the lost structures can be reestablished. Conventional nonsurgical therapy and periodontal flap procedures successfully halt the progression of periodontal disease but result in soft tissue recession that leads to poor esthetics in the anterior dentition. Moreover, conventional periodontal therapy often results in residual pockets usually inaccessible to adequate cleaning, which negatively affect the long-term prognosis of the treated tooth. These compromised outcomes can be avoided or minimized by periodontal regenerative procedures that restore the lost periodontal structures.

Successful periodontal regeneration relies on the re-formation of an epithelial seal, deposition of new acellular extrinsic fiber cementum and insertion of functionally oriented connective tissue fibers into the root surface, and restoration of alveolar bone height.[1] The concept that the cells that repopulate the exposed root surface after periodontal surgery define the nature of the attachment that will form was extensively investigated.[2–6] Therefore, the major factor believed to prevent periodontal regeneration after conventional therapeutic approaches is the migration of epithelial cells into the defect area at a faster rate than that of mesenchymal cells,[7] which leads to the formation of a long junctional epithelium and the prevention of the formation of a new attachment apparatus over the previously diseased root surface.[8–11] Gingival connective tissue cells can also populate the space adjacent to the denuded root surface after conventional periodontal treatment. Repopulation of the exposed root surface by gingival connective tissue cells is speculated to result in the formation of

Department of Periodontics, The University of Texas, Health Science Center at San Antonio, 7703 Floyd Curl Drive, MSC 7894, San Antonio, TX 78229-3900, USA
* Corresponding author.
E-mail address: villar@uthscsa.edu (C.C. Villar).

Dent Clin N Am 54 (2010) 73–92
doi:10.1016/j.cden.2009.08.011
0011-8532/09/$ – see front matter. Published by Elsevier Inc.

dental.theclinics.com

a connective tissue attachment followed by root resorption. Based on this speculation, the goal of regenerative procedures is to prevent apical migration of gingival epithelial and connective tissue cells and to provide maintenance of a wound space into which a selective population of cells (hence guided tissue regeneration [GTR]) is allowed to migrate, favoring the formation of a new periodontal attachment.

BIOLOGIC BASIS OF GTR

GTR has successfully shown to prevent the migration of epithelial and gingival connective tissue cells into previously diseased root surfaces.[11–14] The biologic basis of GTR is based on the assumption that the placement of physical barriers prevents apical migration of the epithelium and gingival connective tissue cells of the flap and provides a secluded space for the inward migration of periodontal ligament cells (PDL) and mesenchymal cells on the exposed root surface,[3] which in turn promote periodontal regeneration. Besides favoring selective repopulation of the wound area, physical barriers are also thought to provide protection of the blood clot during the early phases of healing and to ensure space maintenance for ingrowth of a new periodontal apparatus. GTR membranes, as physical barriers, however, provide no biologic effects on differentiation and proliferation of mesenchymal and PDL cells, which is likely to limit their clinical efficacy.

TYPES OF BARRIER MEMBRANES

Since the discovery that only selected cells have the potential to re-create a new periodontal attachment, a wide range of materials, including methylcellulose acetate, expanded polytetrafluoroethylene (ePTFE) (GORE-TEX, Gore, Flagstaff, AZ, USA), collagen, polyglycoside synthetic polymers, and calcium sulfate were tested for effectiveness and used as a physical barrier in GTR. These membranes are derived from a variety of sources, natural and synthetic, and are either bioabsorbable or nonresorbable.

Nonresorbable Membranes

Nonresorbable membranes, made of methylcellulose acetate (Millipore, Bedford, MA, USA), were successfully used in the first GTR case.[6] However, these membranes were quite fragile and often tended to tear, which limited their clinical use. Methylcellulose acetate barriers were later replaced by nonresorbable ePTFE membranes (GORE-TEX) specifically designed for periodontal regeneration. Most of the current understanding regarding GTR derives from early studies using ePTFE membranes.[15–18]

ePTFE is a synthetic biocompatible polymer consisting of a long carbon backbone to which fluorine atoms are bonded.[19] This membrane is composed of an inner cell occlusive area and an outer cell adherent region.[20] Because of this particular configuration, ePTFE membranes can selectively exclude migration of epithelial and gingival connective tissue cells and integrate with the bone and connective tissue margin of the periodontal defect. This material not only possesses adequate stiffness to allow creation and maintenance of a secluded space into which the new attachment will form[21] but also is supple enough to allow adequate adaptation over the defect. ePTFE membranes are available in various configurations and sizes, in nonreinforced and titanium-reinforced configurations. Titanium-reinforced configurations are specially indicated when the defect anatomy is not supportive, such as in 1-wall defects. Although excellent clinical results have been shown with the use of ePTFE membranes, their use is associated with high frequency of early spontaneous exposure to the oral environment, which compromises their effectiveness.[18] Moreover, these membranes need to be removed after 6 to 8 weeks in a second surgical procedure (**Fig. 1**).

Bioabsorbable Membranes

Bioabsorbable membranes have been developed primarily to avoid a second surgery for membrane removal. Various bioabsorbable materials, including polyglycoside synthetic polymers (ie, polymers of polylactic acid, polyglycolic acid, polylactate/polygalactate), collagen, and calcium sulfate have been frequently used in membrane barriers.[22] Similar to ePTFE membranes, resorbable membranes are biocompatible and exert their function by excluding undesirable cells from migrating into periodontal defects and providing a space for ingrowth of periodontal attachment.[20] The clinical efficacy of bioabsorbable membranes depends on their ability to retain their structural physical integrity during the first 6 to 8 weeks of healing and to be gradually absorbed thereafter. Based on this concept, chemicals and structural modifications (ie, polymerization, cross-linking) were incorporated into bioabsorbable membranes to extend their absorption time and increase the clinical effectiveness of these materials.[23] However, the prolonged collagen resorption rate does not always result in greater periodontal regeneration.[24] It is possible that membranes are only required to maintain their physical integrity for 6 weeks and prolonged retention after that is detrimental to the healing process.

Collagen barrier membranes, made primarily from bovine and porcine type I collagen, were successfully used in the treatment of periodontal defects. Collagen membranes are particularly suitable for GTR applications, as collagen is chemotactic and stimulates proliferation of fibroblasts,[25,26] acts as a barrier for migrating epithelial cells,[23,27,28] provides hemostasis, serves as a fibrillar scaffold for vascular and tissue ingrowth, can be easily shaped, and is readily adaptable. These membranes are resorbed by the enzymatic activity of macrophages and neutrophils.

Degradable polymers constitute a second major group of bioabsorbable barrier membranes. These membranes are formed by copolymerization of polylactic acid, polyglycolic acid, and polylactate/polygalactate. These synthetic membranes remain

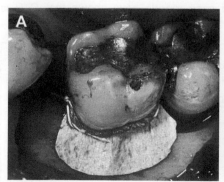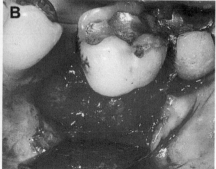

Fig. 1. Treatment of furcation invasion defects with nonresorbable membranes. (*A*) A nonresorbable ePTFE membrane (GORE-TEX) is adapted to cover a furcation defect. (*B*) A second surgical procedure is performed 6 weeks after the initial surgery to remove the nonresorbable membrane. Note the presence of a mature granulation tissue. (*Courtesy of* Michael P. Mills, DMD, MS, University of Texas, Health Science Center at San Antonio, San Antonio, Texas.)

intact for 20 weeks or more, depending on their polymeric composition. Afterward they are degraded by hydrolysis of ester bonds[29] and eliminated through metabolic pathways as carbon dioxide and water. Although these membranes are considered biocompatible, their hydrolysis is accompanied by a local inflammatory response.[21,30] The inflammatory response is not considered harmful, but it remains to be established as to what extent it may affect the regeneration of periodontal tissues.

Calcium sulfate can act as an exclusion barrier and has been used as a GTR membrane in the treatment of periodontal defects. This material provides good adaptation to the margins of the periodontal defect and absorbs in about 30 days[31] without triggering an inflammatory or foreign body reaction.[32,33] Unfortunately, most of the data regarding the use of calcium sulfate in GTR come from either case reports or studies with a relatively small number of cases, in which calcium sulfate was used in association with bone grafting materials, preventing an adequate assessment of its clinical efficacy.

Numerous complications, such as early membrane degradation and epithelial downgrowth, were associated with the use of bioabsorbable barrier membranes. Nevertheless, a meta-analysis of intrabony and furcation defect studies investigating open flap debridement versus GTR revealed that most of the bioabsorbable and nonresorbable GTR membranes provide superior clinical results than open flap debridement alone (**Table 1**).[34] But only a few studies have directly compared the effectiveness of bioabsorbable membranes with open flap debridement as a control. Newer studies comparing the use of bioabsorbable membranes with nonresorbable ePTFE membranes indicate that both membranes are equally effective in the treatment of intrabony and furcation defects.[35–40] The clinical indication of nonresorbable and bioabsorbable membranes necessitates consideration of the anatomy of the periodontal defect. Therefore, nonresorbable reinforced membranes and bioabsorbable membranes supported by filler materials are used for the treatment of nonsupportive defects, such as in wide 1- or 2-walled periodontal defects. On the other hand, narrower 2-walled defects can be treated with bioabsorbable membranes.

CLINICAL OUTCOMES

The clinical efficacy of GTR was reviewed exhaustively. Numerous randomized controlled clinical trials, case series, and case reports have shown that GTR is

Table 1
Additional effect of the use of resorbable or nonresorbable physical barriers as compared with open flap debridement alone in the treatment of intrabony and furcation defects

	Intrabony Defects (mm) (Mean ± SD)		Furcation Defects (mm) (Mean ± SD)		
Barrier	CAL	PD	VPAL	VPD	HOPA
Collagen	0.95 ± 0.47	1.06 ± 0.37	0.1 ± 0.60	−0.04 ± 0.52	0.96 ± 0.91
Polymers	0.92 ± 0.18	0.89 ± 0.14	2.5 ± 0.85	2.30 ± 0.74	Insufficient data
ePTFE	1.62 ± 0.25	1.41 ± 0.2	1.39 ± 0.36	1.01 ± 0.31	0.99 ± 0.31

Abbreviations: CAL, clinical attachment level gain; ePTFE, expanded polytetrafluoroethylene; HOPA, horizontal open probing attachment level gain; PD, probing depth; SD, standard deviation; VPAL, vertical probing attachment level gain; VPD, vertical probing depth reduction.

Data from Murphy KG, Gunsolley JC. Guided tissue regeneration for the treatment of periodontal intrabony and furcation defects. A systematic review. Ann Periodontol 2003;8(1): 266–302.

a successful reconstructive therapeutic option in the management of periodontal intrabony and furcation defects, albeit requiring adequate case selection and excellent surgical skills.

Treatment of Furcation Lesions

The clinical responses of furcation defects to GTR depend on their extent and location. Evidence indicates that GTR can be successfully used only in the treatment of class II mandibular furcations and has a limited clinical effect on class II maxillary furcations.

Class II mandibular furcations

Many randomized clinical trials have addressed the clinical outcomes of GTR in the treatment of class II mandibular furcations.[41–49] A meta-analysis of these studies showed that GTR promotes superior clinical results than flap procedures alone in the treatment of class II mandibular furcations.[50] GTR procedures resulted in significantly greater probing depth reduction when compared with open flap debridement alone (1.16 mm; 95% confidence interval [CI], 0.2–2.52; $P<.001$).[50] Likewise, greater reductions in horizontal furcation depth were observed in sites treated with GTR, weighted mean difference 1.51 mm (95% CI, 0.39–2.62; $P<.001$).[50] Application of barrier membranes consistently and predictably resulted in additional gains in horizontal clinical attachment compared with open flap debridement (1.73 mm; 95% CI, 0.61–2.85; $P<.001$).[50] Although these results clearly indicate an advantage in the use of GTR for the treatment of class II mandibular furcations, complete furcation closure is a rare finding regardless of the treatment used. Additional gains in horizontal clinical attachment associated with GTR procedures allows for the transformation of class II into class I mandibular furcations, which are more easily maintained over time.

Class II maxillary furcations

The clinical effectiveness of GTR in the treatment of class II maxillary furcation defects was investigated in a few randomized controlled clinical trials.[51–53] Meta-analysis of the reported clinical outcomes indicated only a limited added benefit from the placement of barrier membranes after elevation of a flap.[50] For instance, class II maxillary furcation lesions treated with GTR failed to consistently show improved reduction in vertical probing depths when compared with sites treated with open flap debridement alone (mean difference, 1.42 mm; 95% CI, 0.28–2.55; $P = .398$).[50] Also, GTR provided no additional gains in clinical attachment in class II maxillary furcations (0.76 mm; 95% CI, 0.29–1.22; $P = .188$).[50] Although GTR promoted statistically greater reductions in the horizontal furcation depth compared with open flap debridement alone (1.05 mm; 95% CI, 0.46–1.64; $P<.001$),[50] this difference has doubtful clinical significance and does not by itself support the indication of GTR for the treatment of class II maxillary furcations.

Class III furcations

Even though some clinical reports indicate that closure of mandibular class III furcations can be occasionally achieved with GTR,[54,55] the efficacy of GTR in improving or eliminating class III furcations is unpredictable.

Treatment of Intrabony Defects

Data from most randomized controlled clinical trials indicate that treatment of intrabony defects with GTR results in significantly greater probing depth reductions and clinical attachment gains compared with open flap debridement alone.[56–76] The observed differences in favor of GTR are supported by the results of a meta-analysis that shows that compared with open flap debridement, GTR results in an additional gain of

1.22 mm in clinical attachment level (95%CI, 0.80–1.64; P<.001) and further reduction of 2.21 mm in probing depth (95% CI, 0.53–1.88; P<.001).[77] Clinical improvements associated with GTR are independent of the type of barrier membrane used (ie, non-resorbable, resorbable)[35–40] and can be maintained over time.[40]

The predictability of GTR in the treatment of intrabony defects was also addressed. Even though the variability in clinical outcomes obtained with GTR is high, the use of barrier membranes generally provides significant clinical advantages compared with open flap debridement in intrabony defects. A randomized controlled clinical trial showed that the percentage of intrabony defects showing gain in attachment levels was higher after GTR (50.9%) than after conventional flap procedures (33.3%).[72]

FACTORS AFFECTING GTR CLINICAL OUTCOMES

Regeneration of periodontal defects, although possible, is not always a predictable outcome. Several local and patient-related factors may account for the variability in the clinical responses to GTR. To increase the predictability and clinical success of GTR, factors related to the patient, the defect, and the surgical treatment should be evaluated during treatment planning.

Patient Factors Affecting Periodontal Regeneration with GTR

Many patient-related factors may adversely affect the healing outcomes after GTR procedures. Among these factors, smoking,[65,66,78–82] poor plaque control,[80,83–85] and residual periodontal disease actively receive special attention, as these can be controlled through behavioral and therapeutic interventions.

Smoking negatively affects the regenerative outcomes of GTR.[65,66,78–82] Various mechanisms can contribute to the detrimental effects of smoking on healing after GTR, including decreased vascular flow, altered neutrophil function, decreased IgG production and lymphocyte proliferation, impaired fibroblast function, and increased prevalence of periodontal pathogens.[86] The frequency and duration of smoking inversely correlate to clinical attachment gains after GTR. Moreover, a benefit of smoking cessation in patients undergoing GTR has been suggested.[86] However, the time required for host responses to GTR to return to normal after smoking cessation has yet to be determined.

The level of postoperative plaque control and residual periodontal infection, evaluated by the number of residual periodontal pockets and percentage of sites with bleeding on probing, also affects the clinical responses to GTR.[87–89] Barrier membranes are at a higher risk of becoming contaminated in individuals with high levels of periodontal pathogens and multiple sites with bleeding on probing.[87] Therefore, patients should undergo GTR procedures only after periodontal infection has been treated. Ideally, patients should have full mouth plaque and bleeding scores equal to, or lower than, 15% to achieve optimal regenerative outcomes after GTR procedures.[90]

Although there is not enough evidence that diabetes, immunosuppression, and stress impair the efficacy of GTR, it was reported that these patient-related systemic conditions could negatively interfere with the clinical outcomes of GTR.[91]

Local Factors Affecting Periodontal Regeneration with GTR

The predictability of GTR in regenerating the periodontal apparatus is strongly influenced by the local anatomy and morphology of periodontal defects. Case selection is of paramount importance and represents 1 of the most significant factors in predicting the clinical outcomes of GTR procedures.[81,92] The presence of cervical enamel projections and enamel pearls interferes with periodontal regeneration and should be removed during regenerative procedures. The gingival thickness around the affected area should also be analyzed, as gingival thickness less than 1 mm is associated with increased prevalence and severity of flap dehiscence over GTR membranes.[93] Presurgical tooth mobility has a negative effect on the clinical outcome of GTR[72] and should be controlled through splinting and/or occlusal adjustments. Local factors that favor plaque accumulation, such as calculus and overhanging restorations, need to be removed before GTR procedures. In addition to these considerations, specific factors related to the regeneration of furcation and intrabony defects should be evaluated.

Considerations regarding furcation lesions

The predictability and efficacy of GTR procedures in the treatment of furcation lesions are strongly influenced by the tooth anatomy, anatomic features of the furcation area, and morphology of the furcation defect. It was shown that the presence of root concavities could impair the results of GTR, as these concavities prevented adequate membrane adaptation.[94,95] A lack of an intimate adaptation between the barrier membrane and the root surface allows for greater risk of apical migration of the junctional epithelium, thus obviating the barrier function of the membrane and subsequent regeneration. Therefore, when root concavities are present, the collars of barrier membranes should be modified to allow for improved membrane adaptation and clinical results.[94,95] Another important parameter to be considered when evaluating a furcation lesion for GTR is the length of the root trunk. Molars with long root trunks (5–6 mm) show a higher frequency of clinical furcation closure after GTR therapy than molars with short root trunks (≤4 mm).[81] The better prognosis associated with long root might be because coronal positioning of the flap, flap adaptation, and membrane coverage are better achieved in molars with long root trunks.[96]

The clinical success of GTR in furcation defects is strongly affected by the defect morphology. In furcation defects, many aspects of the defect morphology are predictive of the clinical outcomes after GTR.[81] Furcation defects with a horizontal depth of 4 mm or less and small distances between the furcation roof and (a) the base of the defect (4 mm or less), or (b) the crest of the bone (2 mm or less) are associated with improved clinical outcomes.[81] Teeth with interproximal bone heights at the same level or coronal to the roof of the furcation,[81] deep probing pocket depth,[87,89] and narrow root divergence (3 mm or less)[81] exhibit improved clinical outcomes and greater chances of complete furcation closure after GTR.

The regeneration potential of furcation lesions is also dependent on the location of the tooth in the mouth. Evidence indicates that although GTR can be successfully used in the treatment of class II mandibular furcations, it provides only limited advantages in the treatment of class II maxillary furcations.[51] Differences in the clinical outcomes after GTR in maxillary and mandibular furcation defects is likely to be related to the anatomy of the defects, number of roots and furcations, access for root surface debridement, and membrane adaptation.

Considerations regarding intrabony defects

Clinical efficacy of GTR procedures in intrabony defects depends on the morphology of the defect. Clinical evidence indicates that after GTR, intrabony defects deeper than 3 mm show greater probing attachment gain and bone fill than shallow defects.[85,88,97–99] However, the clinical outcome of GTR procedures in shallow and deep defects is similar when probing attachment gains are expressed as a percentage of the baseline intrabony component of the defects.[99]

The width of the intrabony component of the defect, measured by the baseline radiographic angle formed between the bony wall of the defect and long axis of the root,[100] plays an important role in determining the clinical outcomes of GTR. Therefore, narrow defects are consistently associated with increased amounts of probing attachment level gain and bone fill.[88] A quantitative analysis of the effect of the width of the intrabony defects on the clinical outcomes of GTR revealed that intrabony defects with narrow radiographic angles (<25°) gained consistently more attachment than wide defects (>37°).[101] Defect morphology in terms of the number of residual bony walls and tooth surfaces involved was reported to have minimal or no effect on the clinical outcomes of GTR.[85,88] This is surprising, given that the potential for available PDL and mesenchymal cells may differ in different defect morphologies. It is possible that these studies have too low a power to detect differences in clinical outcomes. More studies are warranted to establish the effect of the number of residual bony walls on the clinical outcomes of GTR.

SURGICAL CONSIDERATIONS FOR GTR

After administration of adequate local anesthesia, intrasulcular incisions are placed on the buccal and oral aspects of the defect site, extending at least 1 tooth mesially and distally (**Fig. 2**C). Care should be taken to fully preserve the interproximal soft tissue,[102] as preservation of interproximal gingival tissues is key for optimal defect coverage at wound closure. Several flap designs have been specially designed to preserve the interproximal soft tissue, including the modified and the simplified papilla preservation technique.[57,103–106] Selection of the flap design is primarily based on the width of the interdental space, distance between the contact point and the alveolar bone crest, and location and morphology of the bone defect. The simplified papilla preservation flap is used in areas with a mesiodistal width of the interproximal space greater than 2 mm,[104] and the modified papilla preservation technique is used in narrower interproximal spaces (<2 mm).[103] When a defect is associated with an adjacent edentulous ridge, a crestal incision is performed. Vertical releasing incisions are placed only if necessary for adequate access to the defect site or to achieve complete coverage of the membrane with the mucoperiosteal flap, as vertical incisions compromise vascularization of the flap. Furthermore, all incisions should be placed in areas away from the anticipated membrane placement so that incision lines are not directly over the barrier membrane.

Full-thickness flaps are then elevated to gain adequate visualization and access to the defect and to ensure that the barrier membrane rests on the bone margin adjacent to the defect (see Fig. 2D and Fig. 3C). After flap elevation, the exposed defect is meticulously debrided and the root surfaces scaled and planed (often using a combination of rotating, ultrasonic, and hand instruments) and rinsed with sterile saline solution (see Figs. 2D and 3C). Odontoplasty is performed if required to gain adequate access to the defect and to reduce or eliminate cervical enamel projections or enamel pearls.

The configuration of the defect is then evaluated, and a membrane is selected, trimmed, and adapted over the defect in such a manner that the entire defect and at least 2 to 3 mm of the surrounding alveolar bone is completely covered (see **Figs. 2**E and **3**D, E). Then, if applicable, the barrier is sutured around the neck of the tooth in a tent-like fashion around the root trunk (see **Fig. 3**D, E). Resorbable membranes can either be fixed by using resorbable sutures or simply adapted in place according to the manufacturer's surgical protocol (see **Fig. 2**E). Tenting screws and fixating pins can be used when indicated for membrane stabilization and fixation.

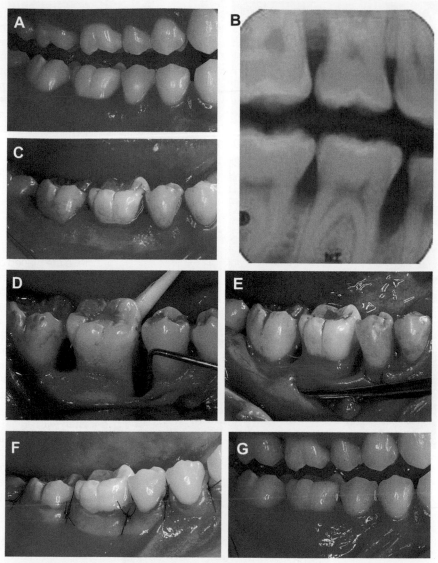

Fig. 2. Treatment of intrabony defects with GTR. (*A*) After scaling and root planning, a 6-mm pocket distal to the lower right second premolar and an 8-mm pocket mesial to the lower right first mandibular molar are evident. (*B*) The pockets are associated with a deep intrabony defect. (*C*) Simplified papilla preservation technique is used to access the defect. Incisions are stopped at the mesial-line angle of the lower right first premolar and at the distal-line angle of the lower right third molar. (*D*) Full-thickness flaps are elevated, and the intrabony defect is seen after debridement. (*E*) A resorbable collagen membrane (Bio-Gide, Osteohealth, Shirley, NY, USA) is sutured around the cementoenamel junction to cover the defect. (*F*) Primary closure of the flaps is achieved with modified vertical internal mattress sutures. (*G*) Excellent early healing with preservation of the interproximal tissue is observed at the 1-week postoperative visit.

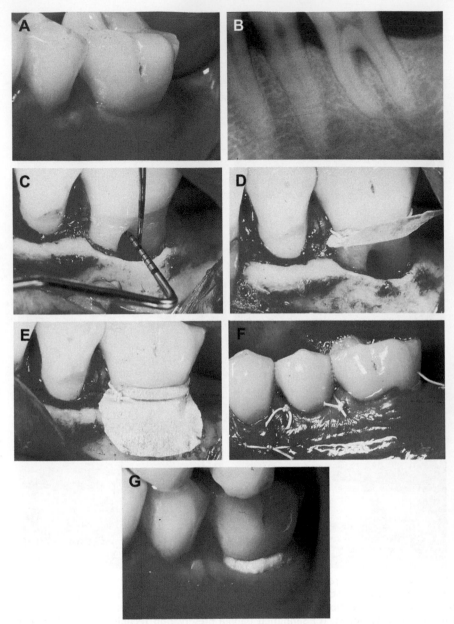

Fig. 3. Treatment of furcation invasion defects with GTR. (*A*) After scaling and root planning, a 2-mm gingival recession and a 7-mm pocket associated with a class II furcation are evident on the facial aspect of the lower left first molar. (*B*) The class II furcation can be radiographically detected. (*C*) Full-thickness flaps are elevated, and the furcation invasion defect is debrided and clinically evaluated. (*D*) A nonresorbable ePTFE membrane (GORE-TEX) is sutured around the cementoenamel junction to cover the defect. For demonstration, the membrane has been lifted off the tooth. (*E*) The membrane is adapted over the defect in such a manner that the entire defect and at least 2 to 3 mm of the surrounding alveolar bone are completely covered. (*F*) Primary closure of the flaps is achieved with simple interrupted ePTFE sutures. (*G*) Membrane exposure is observed at the 4-week postoperative visit. (*Courtesy of* Michael P. Mills, DMD, MS, University of Texas, Health Science Center at San Antonio, San Antonio, Texas.)

Periosteal releasing incisions are made whenever needed to permit tension-free coronal positioning of the flap and complete coverage of the membrane. The mucoperiosteal flaps are repositioned to cover the membrane and then closed with a combination of interrupted and horizontal mattress sutures typically using nonresorbable suture materials (ie, ePTFE), so that the sutures can be left in vivo for periods longer than 7 to 10 days in an effort to maintain wound stability (see Figs. 2F and 3F).

POSTOPERATIVE CARE AND MAINTENANCE

To reduce the risk of postsurgical infection and to ensure optimal clinical results after GTR procedures, systemic antibiotics are generally prescribed. Doxycycline (100 mg orally twice daily) is prescribed for 1 week. Postoperative pain is usually well controlled by nonsteroidal analgesics. Patients are instructed to refrain from mechanical tooth cleaning, including interproximal tooth cleaning, in the surgical site and to rinse twice a day with 0.12% chlorhexidine digluconate for 12 weeks. During the postoperative period, weekly recall visits for monitoring and professional plaque debridment can be helpful. Sutures are generally removed 2 to 3 weeks after surgery. Sutures that loosen prematurely are removed. When using nonresorbable barriers, these membranes should be removed in a second surgical procedure approximately 6 to 8 weeks after their placement. However, if postoperative complications develop, such as membrane exposure, it may be necessary to remove the membrane earlier. Probing and subgingival instrumentation is contraindicated within the first 6 months after surgery.

COMPLICATIONS

Complications associated with GTR procedures are frequent, and they have a negative effect on the clinical outcomes. Membrane exposure constitutes the major complication associated with GTR, with prevalence between 50% and 100%.[18,55,65,82,107-115] The introduction of novel access flaps specifically designed to preserve the interdental tissues[57,103-106] and the use of bioabsorbable membranes have led to a slight reduction in the prevalence of membrane exposure; however, it still constitutes a major complication associated with GTR. Once membrane exposure is clinically detected, efforts should be directed to prevent or treat local infection, as many studies have shown that exposed membranes are contaminated by bacteria[18,89,110,111,113,116-121] and that contaminated membranes are associated with reduced clinical outcomes.[18,110,111,119,120] Depending on the degree of membrane exposure and on the extent of signs of infection near the exposed membrane, exposed membranes should be either removed or treated by a combination of additional systemic antibiotic therapy and topical application of 0.12% chlorhexidine digluconate.[47,118,122,123] Other postoperative complications, including bleeding, swelling, hematoma, erythema, suppuration, sloughing or perforation of the flap, membrane exfoliation, and postoperative pain, have been reported in the immediate postoperative period.[112,124]

COMBINED THERAPY

The placement of bone grafting materials beneath barrier membranes is expected to ensure clot stabilization and space maintenance in nonretentive defects, thereby preventing membrane collapse into the defect. A series of randomized controlled clinical trials have shown that the treatment of class II furcation lesions with barrier membranes with or without the adjunctive use of bone grafts results in significant clinical improvements from baseline.[125-127] Incorporation of bone grafts to GTR procedures in furcation defects results in greater reductions in horizontal probing depths[126,127] when compared with the GTR therapy alone but does not yield significant improvements in other clinical parameters,[125–127] suggesting that it adds a limited value to GTR procedures.

Combined therapy consisting of grafting materials in association with physical barriers was also used in the treatment of periodontal intrabony defects. Despite a limited number of randomized controlled clinical trials evaluating the outcome of combined therapy in the treatment of intrabony defects, the available evidence suggests that incorporation of bone grafts enhances clinical attachment and vertical bone gain in 1-wall intrabony defects treated with barrier membranes.[128] On the other hand, regeneration outcomes obtained from GTR treatment of 2-walled and combined 1-, 2-, and 3-walled intrabony defects are not enhanced by the addition of grafting materials.[129,130] It is likely that incorporation of bone grafts only enhances clinical results in non–self-supporting defects where the incorporation of grafting materials may prevent the collapse of the barrier.

CHALLENGING THE CONCEPT

Successful periodontal regeneration relies on the re-formation of an epithelial seal, deposition of new acellular extrinsic fiber cementum and insertion of functionally oriented connective tissue fibers into the root surface, and restoration of alveolar bone height. The concept that only fibroblasts from the periodontal ligament or undifferentiated mesenchymal cells have the potential to re-create the original periodontal attachment has long been proved. Based on this concept, GTR was applied with variable success to regenerate periodontal defects. However, the quantitative analysis of clinical outcomes after GTR shows that this therapy is indicated only for the treatment of narrow intrabony and class II mandibular defects, suggesting that factors other than the exclusion of the gingival epithelium and connective tissue cells play an important role in periodontal regeneration. It is possible that the spatial relationship established between the bone wall of the defect and the exposed root surface in these 2 types of defects is such that provides a close proximity between the defect and periodontal mesenchymal cell sources allowing for adequate migration and differentiation of these cells into the defect.

Evidence indicates that fibroblast functions, such as migration, proliferation, differentiation, and matrix deposition, strongly depend on their interaction with a growth factor–rich extracellular matrix. Therefore, it is plausible that regeneration of various periodontal defects will only result in a predictable outcome when novel therapeutic approaches that not only prevent migration of undesired cells but also stimulate migration, proliferation, and differentiation of mesenchymal, endothelial, and PDL cells are used. Along these lines, new therapies based on the clinical use of (1) extracellular matrix proteins and angiogenic and cell attachment factors, (2) growth and differentiation factors, (3) biologic mediators of cell metabolism, and (4) stem cells could induce selective cellular repopulation and regeneration of periodontal defects.

SUMMARY

- GTR therapy can be used to treat narrow and deep periodontal intrabony defects. Treatment of intrabony defects with GTR results in significantly greater probing depth reductions and clinical attachment gains compared with open flap debridement alone.

- Although GTR results in significant clinical improvements beyond those achieved with open flap debridement alone in class II mandibular furcations, complete furcation closure is a rare event.
- GTR therapy offers limited clinical benefits in the treatment of class II maxillary furcations and no advantage in the management of class III furcations.
- Nonresorbable and bioabsorbable membranes are equally effective in the treatment of intrabony and class II furcation defects.
- Long-term studies indicate that the clinical gains after GTR can be maintained over time, provided good oral hygiene and appropriate recall programs are maintained.
- It is expected that incorporation of growth and differentiation factors in the GTR treatment of periodontal defects will favor improved clinical results.

REFERENCES

1. Caton JG, Greenstein G. Factors related to periodontal regeneration. Periodontol 2000 1993;1:9–15.
2. Melcher AH. On the repair potential of periodontal tissues. J Periodontol 1976; 47(5):256–60.
3. Gottlow J, Nyman S, Karring T, et al. New attachment formation as the result of controlled tissue regeneration. J Clin Periodontol 1984;11(8):494–503.
4. Gottlow J, Nyman S, Lindhe J, et al. New attachment formation in the human periodontium by guided tissue regeneration. Case reports. J Clin Periodontol 1986;13(6):604–16.
5. Nyman S, Gottlow J, Karring T, et al. The regenerative potential of the periodontal ligament. An experimental study in the monkey. J Clin Periodontol 1982;9(3): 257–65.
6. Nyman S, Lindhe J, Karring T, et al. New attachment following surgical treatment of human periodontal disease. J Clin Periodontol 1982;9(4):290–6.
7. Listgarten MA, Rosenberg MM. Histological study of repair following new attachment procedures in human periodontal lesions. J Periodontol 1979;50(7): 333–44.
8. Bowers GM, Chadroff B, Carnevale R, et al. Histologic evaluation of new attachment apparatus formation in humans. Part I. J Periodontol 1989;60(12):664–74.
9. Caton J, Nyman S, Zander H. Histometric evaluation of periodontal surgery. II. Connective tissue attachment levels after four regenerative procedures. J Clin Periodontol 1980;7(3):224–31.
10. Lindhe J, Nyman S, Karring T. Connective tissue reattachment as related to presence or absence of alveolar bone. J Clin Periodontol 1984;11(1):33–40.
11. Nyman S, Karring T, Lindhe J, et al. Healing following implantation of periodontitis-affected roots into gingival connective tissue. J Clin Periodontol 1980;7(5): 394–401.
12. Karring T, Isidor F, Nyman S, et al. New attachment formation on teeth with a reduced but healthy periodontal ligament. J Clin Periodontol 1985;12(1): 51–60.
13. Karring T, Nyman S, Lindhe J. Healing following implantation of periodontitis affected roots into bone tissue. J Clin Periodontol 1980;7(2):96–105.
14. Melcher AH, McCulloch CA, Cheong T, et al. Cells from bone synthesize cementum-like and bone-like tissue in vitro and may migrate into periodontal ligament in vivo. J Periodont Res 1987;22(3):246–7.

15. Becker W, Becker BE. Treatment of mandibular 3-wall intrabony defects by flap debridement and expanded polytetrafluoroethylene barrier membranes. Long-term evaluation of 32 treated patients. J Periodontol 1993;64(Suppl 11): 1138–44.

16. Flores-de-Jacoby L, Zimmermann A, Tsalikis L. Experiences with guided tissue regeneration in the treatment of advanced periodontal disease. A clinical re-entry study. Part I. Vertical, horizontal and horizontal periodontal defects. J Clin Periodontol 1994;21(2):113–7.

17. Machtei EE, Grossi SG, Dunford R, et al. Long-term stability of Class II furcation defects treated with barrier membranes. J Periodontol 1996;67(5):523–7.

18. Selvig KA, Kersten BG, Chamberlain AD, et al. Regenerative surgery of intrabony periodontal defects using ePTFE barrier membranes: scanning electron microscopic evaluation of retrieved membranes versus clinical healing. J Periodontol 1992;63(12):974–8.

19. Adcock JLI, Shoji, Lagow RJ. Simultaneous fluorination and functionalization of hydrocarbon polymers. J Am Chem Soc 1978;100(6):1948–50.

20. Jovanovic SA, Nevins M. Bone formation utilizing titanium-reinforced barrier membranes. Int J Periodontics Restorative Dent 1995;15(1):56–69.

21. Zellin G, Gritli-Linde A, Linde A. Healing of mandibular defects with different biodegradable and non-biodegradable membranes: an experimental study in rats. Biomaterials 1995;16(8):601–9.

22. Lorenzoni M, Pertl C, Keil C, et al. Treatment of peri-implant defects with guided bone regeneration: a comparative clinical study with various membranes and bone grafts. Int J Oral Maxillofac Implants 1998;13(5):639–46.

23. Minabe M, Kodama T, Kogou T, et al. Different cross-linked types of collagen implanted in rat palatal gingiva. J Periodontol 1989;60(1):35–43.

24. Crigger M, Bogle GC, Garrett S, et al. Repair following treatment of circumferential periodontal defects in dogs with collagen and expanded polytetrafluoroethylene barrier membranes. J Periodontol 1996;67(4):403–13.

25. Locci P, Calvitti M, Belcastro S, et al. Phenotype expression of gingival fibroblasts cultured on membranes used in guided tissue regeneration. J Periodontol 1997;68(9):857–63.

26. Postlethwaite AE, Seyer JM, Kang AH. Chemotactic attraction of human fibroblasts to type I, II, and III collagens and collagen-derived peptides. Proc Natl Acad Sci U S A 1978;75(2):871–5.

27. Kodama T, Minabe M, Hori T, et al. The effect of various concentrations of collagen barrier on periodontal wound healing. J Periodontol 1989;60(4): 205–10.

28. Numabe Y, Ito H, Hayashi H, et al. Epithelial cell kinetics with atelocollagen membranes: a study in rats. J Periodontol 1993;64(8):706–12.

29. Grizzi I, Garreau H, Li S, et al. Hydrolytic degradation of devices based on poly (DL-lactic acid) size-dependence. Biomaterials 1995;16(4):305–11.

30. Zhao S, Pinholt EM, Madsen JE, et al. Histological evaluation of different biodegradable and non-biodegradable membranes implanted subcutaneously in rats. J Craniomaxillofac Surg 2000;28(2):116–22.

31. Bell WH. Resorption characteristics of bone and bone substitutes. Oral Surg Oral Med Oral Pathol 1964;17:650–7.

32. Bahn SL. Plaster: a bone substitute. Oral Surg Oral Med Oral Pathol 1966;21(5): 672–81.

33. Alderman NE. Sterile plaster of paris as an implant in the infrabony environment: a preliminary study. J Periodontol 1969;40(1):11–3.

34. Murphy KG, Gunsolley JC. Guided tissue regeneration for the treatment of peri-odontal intrabony and furcation defects. A systematic review. Ann Periodontol 2003;8(1):266–302.
35. Gottlow J. Guided tissue regeneration using bioresorbable and non-resorbable devices: initial healing and long-term results. J Periodontol 1993;64(Suppl 11): 1157–65.
36. Eickholz P, Kim TS, Holle R. Regenerative periodontal surgery with non-resorb-able and biodegradable barriers: results after 24 months. J Clin Periodontol 1998;25(8):666–76.
37. Caffesse RG, Mota LF, Quinones CR, et al. Clinical comparison of resorbable and non-resorbable barriers for guided periodontal tissue regeneration. J Clin Periodontol 1997;24(10):747–52.
38. Eickholz P, Kim TS, Holle R. Guided tissue regeneration with non-resorbable and biodegradable barriers: 6 months results. J Clin Periodontol 1997;24(2): 92–101.
39. Christgau M, Schmalz G, Reich E, et al. Clinical and radiographical split-mouth-study on resorbable versus non-resorbable GTR-membranes. J Clin Periodontol 1995;22(4):306–15.
40. Kim TS, Holle R, Hausmann E, et al. Long-term results of guided tissue regener-ation therapy with non-resorbable and bioabsorbable barriers. II. A case series of infrabony defects. J Periodontol 2002;73(4):450–9.
41. Wang HL, O'Neal RB, Thomas CL, et al. Evaluation of an absorbable collagen membrane in treating Class II furcation defects. J Periodontol 1994;65(11): 1029–36.
42. Pontoriero R, Lindhe J, Nyman S, et al. Guided tissue regeneration in degree II furcation-involved mandibular molars. A clinical study. J Clin Periodontol 1988; 15(4):247–54.
43. Mombelli A, Zappa U, Bragger U, et al. Systemic antimicrobial treatment and guided tissue regeneration. Clinical and microbiological effects in furcation defects. J Clin Periodontol 1996;23(4):386–96.
44. Lekovic V, Kenney EB, Kovacevic K, et al. Evaluation of guided tissue regener-ation in Class II furcation defects. A clinical re-entry study. J Periodontol 1989; 60(12):694–8.
45. Lekovic V, Kenney EB, Carranza FA, et al. The use of autogenous periosteal grafts as barriers for the treatment of Class II furcation involvements in lower molars. J Periodontol 1991;62(12):775–80.
46. Prathibha PK, Faizuddin M, Pradeep AR. Clinical evaluation of guided tissue regeneration procedure in the treatment of grade II mandibular molar furcations. Indian J Dent Res 2002;13(1):37–47.
47. Cury PR, Sallum EA, Nociti FH Jr, et al. Long-term results of guided tissue re-generation therapy in the treatment of class II furcation defects: a randomized clinical trial. J Periodontol 2003;74(1):3–9.
48. Cury PR, Jeffcoat MK, Sallum AW, et al. Clinical and radiographic evaluation of guided tissue regeneration in the treatment of class II furcation defects. A randomized clinical trial. Spec No. Am J Dent 2003;16:13A–6A.
49. Belal MH, Al-Noamany FA, El-Tonsy MM, et al. Treatment of human class II furca-tion defects using connective tissue grafts, bioabsorbable membrane, and re-sorbable hydroxylapatite: a comparative study. J Int Acad Periodontol 2005; 7(4):114–28.
50. Jepsen S, Eberhard J, Herrera D, et al. A systematic review of guided tissue regeneration for periodontal furcation defects. What is the effect of guided tissue

regeneration compared with surgical debridement in the treatment of furcation defects? J Clin Periodontol 2002;29(Suppl 3):103–16 [discussion: 160–2].

51. Pontoriero R, Lindhe J. Guided tissue regeneration in the treatment of degree II furcations in maxillary molars. J Clin Periodontol 1995;22(10):756–63.

52. Metzler DG, Seamons BC, Mellonig JT, et al. Clinical evaluation of guided tissue regeneration in the treatment of maxillary class II molar furcation invasions. J Periodontol 1991;62(6):353–60.

53. Avera JB, Camargo PM, Klokkevold PR, et al. Guided tissue regeneration in Class II furcation involved maxillary molars: a controlled study of 8 split-mouth cases. J Periodontol 1998;69(9):1020–6.

54. Pontoriero R, Lindhe J, Nyman S, et al. Guided tissue regeneration in the treatment of furcation defects in mandibular molars. A clinical study of degree III involvements. J Clin Periodontol 1989;16(3):170–4.

55. Cortellini P, Pini Prato G, Baldi C, et al. Guided tissue regeneration with different materials. Int J Periodontics Restorative Dent 1990;10(2):136–51.

56. Zucchelli G, Bernardi F, Montebugnoli L, et al. Enamel matrix proteins and guided tissue regeneration with titanium-reinforced expanded polytetrafluoroethylene membranes in the treatment of infrabony defects: a comparative controlled clinical trial. J Periodontol 2002;73(1):3–12.

57. Tonetti MS, Cortellini P, Suvan JE, et al. Generalizability of the added benefits of guided tissue regeneration in the treatment of deep intrabony defects. Evaluation in a multi-center randomized controlled clinical trial. J Periodontol 1998;69(11):1183–92.

58. Silvestri M, Ricci G, Rasperini G, et al. Comparison of treatments of infrabony defects with enamel matrix derivative, guided tissue regeneration with a nonresorbable membrane and Widman modified flap. A pilot study. J Clin Periodontol 2000;27(8):603–10.

59. Sculean A, Windisch P, Chiantella GC, et al. Treatment of intrabony defects with enamel matrix proteins and guided tissue regeneration. A prospective controlled clinical study. J Clin Periodontol 2001;28(5):397–403.

60. Sculean A, Donos N, Schwarz F, et al. Five-year results following treatment of intrabony defects with enamel matrix proteins and guided tissue regeneration. J Clin Periodontol 2004;31(7):545–9.

61. Ratka-Kruger P, Neukranz E, Raetzke P. Guided tissue regeneration procedure with bioresorbable membranes versus conventional flap surgery in the treatment of infrabony periodontal defects. J Clin Periodontol 2000;27(2):120–7.

62. Pritlove-Carson S, Palmer RM, Floyd PD. Evaluation of guided tissue regeneration in the treatment of paired periodontal defects. Br Dent J 1995;179(10):388–94.

63. Pontoriero R, Wennstrom J, Lindhe J. The use of barrier membranes and enamel matrix proteins in the treatment of angular bone defects. A prospective controlled clinical study. J Clin Periodontol 1999;26(12):833–40.

64. Paolantonio M, Perinetti G, Dolci M, et al. Surgical treatment of periodontal intrabony defects with calcium sulfate implant and barrier versus collagen barrier or open flap debridement alone: a 12-month randomized controlled clinical trial. J Periodontol 2008;79(10):1886–93.

65. Mayfield L, Soderholm G, Hallstrom H, et al. Guided tissue regeneration for the treatment of intraosseous defects using a biabsorbable membrane. A controlled clinical study. J Clin Periodontol 1998;25(7):585–95.

66. Loos BG, Louwerse PH, Van Winkelhof AJ, et al. Use of barrier membranes and systemic antibiotics in the treatment of intraosseous defects. J Clin Periodontol 2002;29(10):910–21.

67. Kim CK, Choi EJ, Cho KS, et al. Periodontal repair in intrabony defects treated with a calcium carbonate implant and guided tissue regeneration. J Periodontol 1996;67(12):1301–6.
68. Kilic AR, Efeoglu E, Yilmaz S. Guided tissue regeneration in conjunction with hydroxyapatite-collagen grafts for intrabony defects. A clinical and radiological evaluation. J Clin Periodontol 1997;24(6):372–83.
69. Keles GC, Cetinkaya BO, Isildak I, et al. Levels of platelet activating factor in gingival crevice fluid following periodontal surgical therapy. J Periodont Res 2006;41(6):513–8.
70. Keles GC, Cetinkaya BO, Ayas B, et al. Levels of gingival tissue platelet activating factor after conventional and regenerative periodontal surgery. Clin Oral Investig 2007;11(4):369–76.
71. Joly JC, Palioto DB, de Lima AF, et al. Clinical and radiographic evaluation of periodontal intrabony defects treated with guided tissue regeneration. A pilot study. J Periodontol 2002;73(4):353–9.
72. Cortellini P, Tonetti MS, Lang NP, et al. The simplified papilla preservation flap in the regenerative treatment of deep intrabony defects: clinical outcomes and postoperative morbidity. J Periodontol 2001;72(12):1702–12.
73. Cortellini P, Pini Prato G, Tonetti MS. Periodontal regeneration of human intrabony defects with bioresorbable membranes. A controlled clinical trial. J Periodontol 1996;67(3):217–23.
74. Cortellini P, Pini Prato G, Tonetti MS. Periodontal regeneration of human intrabony defects with titanium reinforced membranes. A controlled clinical trial. J Periodontol 1995;66(9):797–803.
75. Cortellini P, Carnevale G, Sanz M, et al. Treatment of deep and shallow intrabony defects. A multicenter randomized controlled clinical trial. J Clin Periodontol 1998;25(12):981–7.
76. Aimetti M, Romano F, Pigella E, et al. Treatment of wide, shallow, and predominantly 1-wall intrabony defects with a bioabsorbable membrane: a randomized controlled clinical trial. J Periodontol 2005;76(8):1354–61.
77. Needleman IG, Worthington HV, Giedrys-Leeper E, et al. Guided tissue regeneration for periodontal infra-bony defects. Cochrane Database Syst Rev 2006;(2):CD001724.
78. Machtei EE, Schallhorn RG. Successful regeneration of mandibular Class II furcation defects: an evidence-based treatment approach. Int J Periodontics Restorative Dent 1995;15(2):146–67.
79. Machtei EE, Oettinger-Barak O, Peled M. Guided tissue regeneration in smokers: effect of aggressive anti-infective therapy in Class II furcation defects. J Periodontol 2003;74(5):579–84.
80. Tonetti MS, Pini-Prato G, Cortellini P. Effect of cigarette smoking on periodontal healing following GTR in infrabony defects. A preliminary retrospective study. J Clin Periodontol 1995;22(3):229–34.
81. Bowers GM, Schallhorn RG, McClain PK, et al. Factors influencing the outcome of regenerative therapy in mandibular Class II furcations: part I. J Periodontol 2003;74(9):1255–68.
82. Trombelli L, Kim CK, Zimmerman GJ, et al. Retrospective analysis of factors related to clinical outcome of guided tissue regeneration procedures in intrabony defects. J Clin Periodontol 1997;24(6):366–71.
83. Cortellini P, Pini-Prato G, Tonetti M. Periodontal regeneration of human infrabony defects (V). Effect of oral hygiene on long-term stability. J Clin Periodontol 1994;21(9):606–10.

84. Cortellini P, Stalpers G, Pini Prato G, et al. Long-term clinical outcomes of abutments treated with guided tissue regeneration. J Prosthet Dent 1999;81(3): 305–11.
85. Tonetti MS, Prato GP, Cortellini P. Factors affecting the healing response of intrabony defects following guided tissue regeneration and access flap surgery. J Clin Periodontol 1996;23(6):548–56.
86. Johnson GK, Hill M. Cigarette smoking and the periodontal patient. J Periodontol 2004;75(2):196–209.
87. Nowzari H, MacDonald ES, Flynn J, et al. The dynamics of microbial colonization of barrier membranes for guided tissue regeneration. J Periodontol 1996;67(7): 694–702.
88. Tonetti MS, Pini-Prato G, Cortellini P. Periodontal regeneration of human intrabony defects. IV. Determinants of healing response. J Periodontol 1993;64(10):934–40.
89. Machtei EE, Cho MI, Dunford R, et al. Clinical, microbiological, and histological factors which influence the success of regenerative periodontal therapy. J Periodontol 1994;65(2):154–61.
90. Cortellini P. Reconstructive periodontal surgery: a challenge for modern periodontology. Int Dent J 2006;56(4 Suppl 1):250–5.
91. Mattson JS, Gallagher SJ, Jabro MH, et al. Complications associated with diabetes mellitus after guided tissue regeneration: case report. Compend Contin Educ Dent 1998;19(9):923–6, 928, 930 passim; quiz 938.
92. Cortellini P, Tonetti MS. Focus on intrabony defects: guided tissue regeneration. Periodontol 2000 2000;22:104–32.
93. Anderegg CR, Martin SJ, Gray JL, et al. Clinical evaluation of the use of decalcified freeze-dried bone allograft with guided tissue regeneration in the treatment of molar furcation invasions. J Periodontol 1991;62(4):264–8.
94. Novaes AB Jr, Tamani JP, Oliveira PT, et al. Root trunk concavities as a risk factor for regenerative procedures of class II furcation lesions in dogs. J Periodontol 2001;72(5):612–9.
95. Villaca JH, Rodrigues DC, Novaes AB Jr, et al. Root trunk concavities as a risk factor for regenerative procedures of class II furcation lesions in humans. J Periodontol 2004;75(11):1493–9.
96. Hutchens LH Jr. Hypothetical considerations in the regenerative treatment of molar furcation defects. Curr Opin Periodontol 1996;3:157–67.
97. Laurell L, Gottlow J, Zybutz M, et al. Treatment of intrabony defects by different surgical procedures. A literature review. J Periodontol 1998;69(3):303–13.
98. Garrett S, Loos B, Chamberlain D, et al. Treatment of intraosseous periodontal defects with a combined adjunctive therapy of citric acid conditioning, bone grafting, and placement of collagenous membranes. J Clin Periodontol 1988; 15(6):383–9.
99. Cortellini P, Clauser C, Prato GP. Histologic assessment of new attachment following the treatment of a human buccal recession by means of a guided tissue regeneration procedure. J Periodontol 1993;64(5):387–91.
100. Steffensen B, Webert HP. Relationship between the radiographic periodontal defect angle and healing after treatment. J Periodontol 1989;60(5):248–54.
101. Cortellini PT, Tonetti MS. Radiographic defect angle influences the outcomes of GTR therapy in intrabony defects. 77th General Session of the IADR. Vancouver: Canada; 1999.
102. Nygaard-Ostby P, Tellefsen G, Sigurdsson TJ, et al. Periodontal healing following reconstructive surgery: effect of guided tissue regeneration. J Clin Periodontol 1996;23(12):1073–9.

103. Cortellini P, Prato GP, Tonetti MS. The modified papilla preservation technique. A new surgical approach for interproximal regenerative procedures. J Periodontol 1995;66(4):261–6.
104. Cortellini P, Prato GP, Tonetti MS. The simplified papilla preservation flap. A novel surgical approach for the management of soft tissues in regenerative procedures. Int J Periodontics Restorative Dent 1999;19(6):589–99.
105. Cortellini P, Pini Prato G, Tonetti MS. The modified papilla preservation technique with bioresorbable barrier membranes in the treatment of intrabony defects. Case reports. Int J Periodontics Restorative Dent 1996;16(6):546–59.
106. Murphy KG. Interproximal tissue maintenance in GTR procedures: description of a surgical technique and 1-year reentry results. Int J Periodontics Restorative Dent 1996;16(5):463–77.
107. Becker W, Becker BE, Berg L, et al. New attachment after treatment with root isolation procedures: report for treated Class III and Class II furcations and vertical osseous defects. Int J Periodontics Restorative Dent 1988;8(3):8–23.
108. Cortellini P, Pini Prato G, Tonetti MS. Periodontal regeneration of human infrabony defects. I. Clinical measures. J Periodontol 1993;64(4):254–60.
109. Zucchelli G, Bernardi F, Montebugnoli L, et al. Early bacterial accumulation on guided tissue regeneration membrane materials. An in vivo study. J Periodontol 1998;69(11):1193–202.
110. De Sanctis M, Zucchelli G, Clauser C. Bacterial colonization of barrier material and periodontal regeneration. J Clin Periodontol 1996;23(11):1039–46.
111. De Sanctis M, Zucchelli G, Clauser C. Bacterial colonization of bioabsorbable barrier material and periodontal regeneration. J Periodontol 1996;67(11): 1193–200.
112. Murphy KG. Postoperative healing complications associated with Gore-Tex Periodontal Material. Part I. Incidence and characterization. Int J Periodontics Restorative Dent 1995;15(4):363–75.
113. Selvig KA, Kersten BG, Wikesjo UM. Surgical treatment of intrabony periodontal defects using expanded polytetrafluoroethylene barrier membranes: influence of defect configuration on healing response. J Periodontol 1993;64(8):730–3.
114. Tsitoura E, Tucker R, Suvan J, et al. Baseline radiographic defect angle of the intrabony defect as a prognostic indicator in regenerative periodontal surgery with enamel matrix derivative. J Clin Periodontol 2004;31(8):643–7.
115. Falk H, Laurell L, Ravald N, et al. Guided tissue regeneration therapy of 203 consecutively treated intrabony defects using a bioabsorbable matrix barrier. Clinical and radiographic findings. J Periodontol 1997;68(6):571–81.
116. Grevstad HJ, Leknes KN. Ultrastructure of plaque associated with polytetrafluoroethylene (PTFE) membranes used for guided tissue regeneration. J Clin Periodontol 1993;20(3):193–8.
117. Mombelli A, Lang NP, Nyman S. Isolation of periodontal species after guided tissue regeneration. J Periodontol 1993;64(Suppl 11):1171–5.
118. Novaes AB Jr, Gutierrez FG, Francischetto IF, et al. Bacterial colonization of the external and internal sulci and of cellulose membranes at time of retrieval. J Periodontol 1995;66(10):864–9.
119. Nowzari H, Matian F, Slots J. Periodontal pathogens on polytetrafluoroethylene membrane for guided tissue regeneration inhibit healing. J Clin Periodontol 1995;22(6):469–74.
120. Nowzari H, Slots J. Microorganisms in polytetrafluoroethylene barrier membranes for guided tissue regeneration. J Clin Periodontol 1994;21(3): 203–10.

121. Tempro PJ, Nalbandian J. Colonization of retrieved polytetrafluoroethylene membranes: morphological and microbiological observations. J Periodontol 1993;64(3):162–8.
122. Newman MG. The role of infection and anti-infection treatment in regenerative therapy. J Periodontol 1993;64(Suppl 11):1166–70.
123. Bouchard P, Giovannoli JL, Mattout C, et al. Clinical evaluation of a bioabsorbable regenerative material in mandibular class II furcation therapy. J Clin Periodontol 1997;24(7):511–8.
124. Murphy KG. Postoperative healing complications associated with Gore-Tex Periodontal Material. Part II. Effect of complications on regeneration. Int J Periodontics Restorative Dent 1995;15(6):548–61.
125. Wallace SC, Gellin RG, Miller MC, et al. Guided tissue regeneration with and without decalcified freeze-dried bone in mandibular Class II furcation invasions. J Periodontol 1994;65(3):244–54.
126. De Leonardis D, Garg AK, Pedrazzoli V, et al. Clinical evaluation of the treatment of class II furcation involvements with bioabsorbable barriers alone or associated with demineralized freeze-dried bone allografts. J Periodontol 1999; 70(1):8–12.
127. Simonpietri CJ, Novaes AB Jr, Batista EL Jr, et al. Guided tissue regeneration associated with bovine-derived anorganic bone in mandibular class II furcation defects. 6-month results at re-entry. J Periodontol 2000;71(6):904–11.
128. Paolantonio M. Combined periodontal regenerative technique in human intrabony defects by collagen membranes and anorganic bovine bone. A controlled clinical study. J Periodontol 2002;73(2):158–66.
129. Stavropoulos A, Karring ES, Kostopoulos L, et al. Deproteinized bovine bone and gentamicin as an adjunct to GTR in the treatment of intrabony defects: a randomized controlled clinical study. J Clin Periodontol 2003;30(6):486–95.
130. Trejo PM, Weltman R, Caffesse R. Treatment of intraosseous defects with bioabsorbable barriers alone or in combination with decalcified freeze-dried bone allograft: a randomized clinical trial. J Periodontol 2000;71(12):1852–61.

Periodontal Regeneration: Focus on Growth and Differentiation Factors

Jaebum Lee, DDS, MSc, PhD[a], Andreas Stavropoulos, DDS, PhD[b],
Cristiano Susin, DDS, MSD, PhD[a], Ulf M.E. Wikesjö, DDS, DMD, PhD[a],*

KEYWORDS

- Periodontal regeneration • Growth factors
- Differentiation factors • Preclinical study

The periodontium encompasses the alveolar bone, root cementum, periodontal ligament (PDL), and gingiva, which are the tissues surrounding and supporting the teeth. Periodontitis is an inflammatory disease characterized by destruction of the alveolar bone, root cementum, PDL, and gingiva as a response to insults elicited by microbial accumulations on tooth surfaces. Regeneration is defined as the reproduction or reconstitution of a lost or injured part, with form and function of lost structures restored.[1] Periodontal regeneration includes regeneration of alveolar bone, cementum, PDL, and gingiva.

Periodontal defects may be morphologically characterized as suprabony or intrabony, as furcation or gingival recession defects, or their combinations. Defect configuration appears to be one important factor that may predict outcomes of periodontal reconstructive and regenerative procedures. The spatial distribution of vascular and cellular tissue elements circumscribing the defect plays an important role for the healing of any periodontal defect. These tissue elements, which have periodontal or alveolar origin, are dramatically reduced in two- and one-wall intrabony defects, class II and III furcation defects, and in supra-alveolar defects. Accordingly, the number of bone walls and adjoining periodontal tissues appears to be a critical determinant to treatment outcomes[2] in clinical settings. This means that supra-alveolar periodontal defects have significantly reduced potential for regeneration.

[a] Laboratory for Applied Periodontal & Craniofacial Regeneration (LAPCR), Departments of Periodontics and Oral Biology, Medical College of Georgia School of Dentistry, 1120 5th Street AD1434, Augusta, GA 30912, USA
[b] Department of Periodontology, University of Aarhus School of Dentistry, Vennelyst Boulevard 9, DK-8000, Aarhus C, Denmark
* Corresponding author.
E-mail address: uwikesjo@mail.mcg.edu (U.M.E. Wikesjö).

Dent Clin N Am 54 (2010) 93–111
doi:10.1016/j.cden.2009.09.001
0011-8532/09/$ – see front matter © 2010 Elsevier Inc. All rights reserved.

dental.theclinics.com

Animal models are useful for observing the nature of wound healing following periodontal regenerative therapy, and for evaluating the efficacy and safety of biomaterials, devices, and biologic factors included in surgical protocols to support or induce periodontal regeneration before such protocols are applied clinically. Animal studies have been performed using rodent, feline, porcine, caprine, ovine, canine, and nonhuman primate models. Variations among species including, but not limited to, anatomy and dimensions of teeth and alveolar processes, amount and character of the gingiva, local physiologic environment, animal behavior, and healing rate make each animal model unique. None of the species listed provide an anatomic and physiologic environment equal to the human oral cavity. However, dogs, which are skeletally larger and easier to handle than many of the other animal models, are preferred for study of periodontal wound healing and regeneration because their physiology is reasonably close to that of humans, they have a clinically relevant size and tooth configuration, they are significantly easier to handle than most other animals during essential postoperative management, and they are the subjects of extensive published research experience. Many other species, including nonhuman primates, may not be as useful in oral wound healing studies because of difficulties in gaining access for required postsurgery follow-up and, especially in the case of nonhuman primates, because of their ability to perturb surgical sites.

Several animal models and defect types have been proposed in the literature for the study of periodontal wound healing and regeneration. Wikesjö and colleagues[3] developed and characterized supracrestal periodontal defects into a critical-size defect model. The model comprises surgically created, circumferential, supra-alveolar periodontal defects, 5 to 6 mm in height (from the cementoenamel junction to the reduced alveolar crest) around the mandibular third and fourth premolar teeth in dogs. Through various experimental studies, this critical-size, supra-alveolar, periodontal defect model has been proven to be a discriminating tool, a "litmus test," for the preclinical evaluation of candidate therapies for periodontal wound healing and regeneration, including therapies involving bone biomaterials, devices for guided tissue regeneration, growth and differentiation factors, and their combinations. Significant regeneration in this challenging model warrants clinical evaluation of the therapeutic concept; conversely, limited regeneration under optimal circumstances for wound healing does not warrant clinical follow-up.

This article reviews studies evaluating growth and differentiation factors considered candidate therapeutic agents for periodontal wound healing/regeneration. The article focuses on studies using relevant preclinical models and pivotal clinical trials where available. These studies support a rationale for the clinical evaluation and eventual use of a number of growth and differentiation factors to enhance or secure outcomes following regenerative procedures in periodontal defects.

GROWTH FACTORS

Regeneration of periodontal structures constitutes a complex multifactor process regulated by interactions among cells, hormones, growth factors, and extracellular matrices. These interactions trigger a series of events leading to de novo tissue formation. This process is still incompletely understood. However, advances in molecular and cellular biology have contributed to an understanding of the potential role of growth factors in periodontal wound healing and regeneration and their use as therapeutic agents. Several matrix, growth, and differentiation factors have received attention because of their ability to actively regulate various functions of PDL cells. The effects of such factors as they apply to periodontal regeneration have been evaluated.

Examples of growth factors associated with periodontal tissues and considered as candidate agents in support of periodontal wound healing or regeneration include platelet-derived growth factor (PDGF), insulinlike growth factors I and II (IGF-I and -II), acidic and basic fibroblast growth factors (aFGF and bFGF), and transforming growth factor β (TGF-β) **(Table 1)**.

Platelet-Derived Growth Factor

PDGF, a polypeptide growth factor, has potent stimulatory effects as a chemoattractant and mitogen for mesenchymal cells (including osteogenic cells), along with an ability to promote angiogenesis in wound healing.[26] The PDGF family includes four isoforms: PDGF-A, PDGF-B, and recently discovered PDGF-C and PDGF-D.[27,28] PDGF-A and -B are both present in gingival epithelium. PDGF-A may have a prominent role during early wound healing, while PDGF-B may regulate later events.[29] PDGF-A and -B form homodimers (AA or BB) and a heterodimer (AB). In vitro, studies have demonstrated that all three forms enhance gingival and PDL fibroblast chemotaxis, proliferation, and protein synthesis,[30-33] with PDGF-BB apparently being the most effective ligand.[31,34] PDGF-BB application onto surface demineralized dentin has been shown to stimulate human PDL cell proliferation[35] and increase cementoblast mitogenesis in vitro.[36,37] Moreover, PDGF-BB stimulates human PDL cell proliferation and collagen synthesis in a time- and dose-dependent order reaching maximum effect at 24 hours at a dose of 10 ng/mL.[33]

The effect of PDGF in a carrier or combined with guided tissue regeneration (GTR) has been evaluated in periodontal fenestration defects in dogs.[4] Autoradiography showed significantly increased fibroblast proliferation following PDGF application compared with GTR or sham-surgery controls at 1 and 7 days postsurgery. In other studies using chronic class III furcation defects in dogs, a PDGF-BB/GTR/root surface demineralization protocol apparently produced favorable periodontal regeneration compared with the carrier control.[5,6] Nonhuman primate periodontal defects implanted with PDGF-BB showed significantly greater new attachment formation and bone fill compared with vehicle control at 12 weeks postsurgery.[7] In summary, in vitro studies suggest that PDGF-BB exerts several important effects on cells native to the periodontal environment; and in vivo preclinical studies suggest that PDGF-BB exerts stimulatory effects on periodontal wound healing and regeneration, thus motivating clinical follow-up.

A multicenter phase III randomized controlled clinical trial assessed the safety and efficacy of recombinant human PDGF-BB (rhPDGF-BB) in a β-tricalcium phosphate (β-TCP) carrier.[8] One hundred-eighty subjects requiring surgical treatment of 4-mm or deeper intrabony periodontal defects were randomized to receive rhPDGF-BB at 0.3 or 1.0 mg/mL, or carrier control. Clinical and radiographic evaluations were performed presurgery, and at 3 and 6 months postsurgery. No serious adverse effects attributable to treatments were recorded. Significantly improved attachment levels were observed for sites receiving rhPDGF-BB at 0.3 mg/mL compared with control at 3 months; however, the mean effect was limited (ie, 3.8 vs 3.3 mm). There were no significant differences in attachment level gain at 6 months, attachment level gain averaging 3.8 versus 3.5 mm, respectively. Compared with control or rhPDGF-BB at 0.3 mg/mL, rhPDGF-BB at 1.0 mg/mL exhibited no remarkable or significant differences. A biopsy study including intrabony periodontal in eight patients treated with rhPDGF-BB at 0.3 or 1.0 mg/mL in the β-TCP carrier showed limited periodontal regeneration in 12 of 16 defects (range 0.3–1.6 mm) following a 6-month or greater healing interval.[9] Bone formation never juxtaposed new cementum formation. A majority of the defect sites were filled with residual β-TCP, with bone formation never penetrating the β-TCP

Table 1
Effect of growth factors on periodontal wound healing/regeneration in preclinical models and pivotal clinical studies.

Factor (Preclinical or Clinical)	Model; Platform	Dose; Carrier; Healing Interval	Major Observation	References
PDGF (preclinical)	Fenestration; dog	10 µg/mL; topical application; 1, 3, 7d	Increased fibroblast proliferation	4
	Class III furcation; dog	0.5 µg/mL; topical application; 5, 8, 11 wk	Favorable periodontal regeneration including bone fill	5,6
	Chronic periodontitis; nonhuman primate	10 µg; methylcellulose gel; 4, 12 wk	Increased new attachment and bone fill	7
PDGF (clinical)	Phase III randomized controlled trial, 180 patients, ≥4-mm intrabony defects; clinical	0.3, 1.0 mg/mL; β-TCP; 3, 6 mo	0.3 mg/mL: improved attachment level at 3 mo; 1.0 mg/mL: not different from control	8
	Case series, 8 patients, defects; clinical and biopsies	0.3, 1.0 mg/mL; β-TCP; 6 mo	Limited periodontal regeneration	9
IGF (preclinical)	Chronic periodontitis; nonhuman primate	10 µg; methylcellulose gel; 4, 12 wk	No periodontal regeneration	7
FGF (preclinical)	3-wall intrabony; dog	30, 40, 50 µg; fibrin gel; 6 wk	Dose-dependent periodontal regeneration	10
	2-3 wall intrabony and class II furcation; nonhuman primate	30, 40, 50 µg; fibrin gel; 8 wk	Dose-dependent periodontal regeneration	10
	Class II furcation; dog	30 µg; topical application; 6 wk	Increased PDL, bone formation	11
	Class II furcation; nonhuman primate	0.1%, 0.4%; gelatin; 8 wk	Dose-dependent bone and cement regeneration	12
	Class III furcation; dog	0.5, 1.0 mg; topical application; 90 d	Low dose: greater cement and bone formation	13
	Reimplanted incisor; dog	0.1, 1,5 µg; collagen gel; 4, 8 wk	Enhanced cementum formation, PDL fiber	14

FGF (clinical)	Phase II randomized controlled trial, 74 patients, 2–3 wall intrabony defects; clinical	0.03%, 0.1%, 0.3%; hydroxypropyl cellulose; 9 mo	Enhanced alveolar bone height, PDL regeneration	15
TGF-β (preclinical)	Class II furcation; sheep	80 µg/mL; 25% pluronic F-127; 6 wk	TGF-β1 plus GTR enhanced bone formation over TGF-β1 alone	16
	Supra-alveolar; dog	20 µg; calcium carbonate composite; 4 wk	Limited cementum and bone formation	17–21
	Class II furcation; nonhuman primate	1.5, 2.5 µg; gelatinous, heterotopic induced ossicles, minced muscle tissue; 8 wk	Enhanced vascularity, substantial regeneration	22
RhPDGF-B/IGF-1 (preclinical)	Periodontitis defects; dog	1/1 µg; aqueous gel; 2, 5 wk	Enhanced bone and cementum formation	23,24
	Chronic intrabony defects; nonhuman primate	10/10 µg; methylcellulose gel; 4, 12 wk	Greater periodontal regeneration	7
RhPDGF-B/IGF-1 (clinical)	Phase I/II randomized controlled trial, 38 patients, bilateral intrabony and furcation defects; clinical	50/50, 150/150 µg/mL; gel; 6, 9 mo	150/150 µg/mL rhPDGF-BB/IGF-1 dose increased bone fill	25

Abbreviations: β-TCP, β-tricalcium phosphate; GTR, guided tissue regeneration; rhPDGF-B recombinant human PDGF-B mass or contacting the particles. The unremarkable clinical and histologic improvements noted following rhPDGF-BB treatment in these studies raises questions about the relevance and utility of this treatment modality in patient-centered settings.

Insulinlike Growth Factors

IGF-1 and -2 play a critical role in stimulating organogenesis and growth during early stages of embryogenesis as well as in regulation of specific tissue and organ functions at later stages of development.[38,39] IGF-1 affects cementoblast mitogenesis, phenotypic gene expression, and mineralization[37]; and stimulates bone formation,[40–42] growth,[43] and resorption.[44] In vitro, IGF-1 enhances rat and human PDL and gingival fibroblast migration and proliferation in a dose and temporal order, but IGF-1 does not exhibit an apparent effect on type I collagen synthesis.[31,45,46] These observations suggest that IGF-1 might play a role in periodontal wound healing and regeneration.

Preclinical studies using IGF-1 in a methylcellulose gel carrier, however, failed to show regeneration of the periodontal attachment following application into induced nonhuman primate chronic periodontal defects.[7] Incremental increases in osteoblast numbers and bone formation compared with sham-surgery control were reported in canine periodontitis defects implanted with IGF-1.[47] Collectively the results may be interpreted to suggest that IGF-1 has limited, if any, appreciable effects on periodontal wound healing or regeneration.

Fibroblast Growth Factor

FGFs exert a range of biologic effects on cells of endodermal, ectodermal, and mesodermal origin; are considered potent growth and differentiation regulators and angiogenic factors; and play important roles in development and wound healing. BFGF (also called FGF-2) found in bone matrix[48,49] is a multifunctional factor that induces proliferation and morphogenesis in a wide range of cells and tissues, including the PDL.[14] BFGF also appears to exert profound effects on bone growth and development,[50,51] and enhances fracture healing.[52] Moreover, bFGF inhibits alkaline phosphatase activity and PDL cell mineralized nodule formation in vitro.[10]

Surgically created three-wall intrabony defects implanted with bFGF at various dosages exhibited significantly greater periodontal regeneration compared with carrier or sham-surgery controls at 6 weeks in dogs and at 8 weeks in nonhuman primates.[10] The high dose generated an approximately twofold increase in cementum and bone formation regardless of the species used for testing. Epithelial down growth or root resorption/ankylosis were not observed. In a second study, topical application of rhbFGF (30 μg/site) in a gelatinous carrier into surgically created class II furcation defects in dogs induced increased PDL, cementum, and bone formation compared with control at 6 weeks.[11] Dose-dependent periodontal regeneration was observed at 8 weeks in nonhuman primates using 0.1% or 0.4% rhbFGF with the gelatinous carrier; the high-dose group showed significant bone and cementum regeneration.[12] The effect of bFGF (0.5 or 1.0 mg/site) combined with GTR on periodontal wound healing/regeneration was analyzed in surgically induced mandibular premolar class III furcation defects in dogs.[13] Test sites received bFGF after root conditioning with tetracycline hydrochloride (HCl). Increased regeneration was observed in sites receiving bFGF compared with control at 90 days. Notably, the low-dose group exhibited greater cementum and bone formation compared with the high-dose group. Root resorption/ankylosis was not observed. In yet another study, cementum formation was enhanced following application of bFGF (0.1, 1, and 5 μg/site) in a collagen gel into dentinal defects in freshly extracted and then reimplanted mandibular incisors in dogs.[14] Random PDL fibers attached to dentin were observed at 4 weeks. Newly synthesized dense fibers invading alveolar bone and cementum were observed at 8 weeks in the 1-µg bFGF group. In vitro and in vivo preclinical observations justified the need for clinical trials to determine the potential of bFGF to promote periodontal regeneration also in humans.

A randomized controlled phase II clinical trial enrolled 74 patients with two- or three-wall intrabony periodontal defects to evaluate the effect of rhbFGF in a hydroxypropylcellulose gel carrier on periodontal wound healing/regeneration.[15] A significant increase in alveolar bone height was noted after 36 weeks, suggesting that rhbFGF stimulates regeneration of the PDL also in humans. Taken together, the studies suggest that bFGF may serve as a useful therapeutic adjunct to surgical procedures aimed at promoting periodontal wound healing and regeneration.

Transforming Growth Factor–β

TGF-β stimulates PDL cell extracellular matrix synthesis, mitogenesis, and proliferation.[30,31,45] TGF-β receptors are up-regulated in regenerated PDL tissues, suggesting that TGF-β may also be capable of mediating periodontal regeneration.[53]

TGF-β_1 at 80 µg/mL in a gelatinous carrier, 25% Pluronic F-127 (poloxamer 407), and TGF-β_1 in the gelatinous carrier combined with GTR were implanted into surgically created, mandibular premolar class II furcation defects in sheep. Significantly, enhanced bone formation was demonstrated for TGF-β_1 compared with carrier control at 6 weeks; the TGF-β_1/GTR combination significantly enhanced bone formation over TGF-β_1 alone.[16] Contrasting results were reported in studies using the canine critical-size, supra-alveolar periodontal defect model.[17–21] Using a split-mouth design and a 4-week healing interval, contralateral defects in six animals received rhTGF-β_1 (20 µg/defect) in a calcium carbonate ($CaCO_3$) composite carrier versus carrier control, both combined with GTR. Defects in another six animals received rhTGF-β_1 versus carrier control without GTR, and still another six animals received carrier control combined with GTR versus GTR without additions. The histometric analysis showed limited, if any, cementum regeneration, without obvious differences between experimental groups, and bone formation generally limited to the apical aspect of the defects. Collectively, the results from these studies suggest that TGF-β_1 possesses a clinically insignificant, if any, potential to stimulate periodontal wound healing or regeneration. Other studies suggest that TGF-β_3 may enhance periodontal wound healing/regeneration.[22] Surgically created class II furcation defects in nonhuman primates, implanted with TGF-β_3 in a Matrigel carrier (a gelatinous protein mixture), TGF-β_3 plus carrier plus heterotopic TGF-β_3–induced ossicles, TGF-β_3 plus carrier plus minced muscle tissue, or carrier alone showed pronounced regeneration in TGF-β_3–implanted sites compared with controls at 8 weeks. Striking vascularization in sites receiving TGF-β_3 and displaying multiple capillaries along the edge of the alveolar bone appeared to preside insertion of Sharpey fibers. Notably, substantial regeneration was observed in defects implanted with heterotopically TGF-β_3–induced ossicles and with TGF-β_3 plus minced muscle tissue. A clinical follow-up of a TGF-β_3–based therapy appears to be not yet available. Unfortunately, the use of ad hoc defect models without thorough characterization makes the results difficult to interpret and compare with those from established discriminating critical-size defect models, which is why these promising observations also need to be confirmed in such established models.

Growth Factor Combinations

Combinations of growth factors might be used to synergistically improve periodontal wound healing/regeneration. Most investigators have evaluated the effects of single factors only and might thus have overlooked potential large biologic responses comparable with those documented in the literature when growth factors used in combinations interact synergistically in vitro. For example, combinations of PDGF-BB, IGF-1, and TGF-β_1 stimulated PDL cell mitogenesis and adhesion.[54–56] Interactions among IGF-1, PDGF-BB, TGF-β_1, and bFGF were evaluated in other studies. Fetal bovine osteoblasts were assessed for surrogates of bone formation and metabolism/remodeling, including osteoblast mitogenesis, collagenous and noncollagenous protein synthesis, and alkaline phosphatase activity. Even though synergistic interactions between IGF-1 and the other factors relative to osteoblast mitogenic activity and protein synthesis were observed, IGF-1 failed to increase alkaline phosphatase activity when combined with TGF-β_1, PDGF-BB, and bFGF.[55]

An rhPDGF-B/IGF-1 construct surgically implanted into periodontitis defects in dogs significantly increased bone and cementum formation compared with control following a 2- and 5-week healing interval.[23,24] In a parallel study using nonhuman primates, induced chronic intrabony defects were implanted with rhPDGF-B/IGF-I, rhPDGF-B, rhIGF-1, or carrier control.[7] Significantly greater periodontal regeneration was observed in sites receiving the rhPDGF-B/IGF-1 combination compared with individual factors or the carrier control following 4 and 12 weeks.

The positive in vitro and in vivo preclinical evaluation of the rhPDGF-B/IGF-1 combination motivated a clinical evaluation. Thirty-eight patients with bilateral intrabony and furcation defects participated in a phase I/II clinical trial.[25] Defect sites received surgical implantation of rhPDGF-BB/IGF-I (50 or 150 μg/mL each) in a gel carrier, and were compared with carrier control or sham surgery. Bone fill was evaluated using surgical reentry at 6 to 9 months postsurgery. Subjects receiving the rhPDGF-BB/IGF-I (50/50 μg/mL) combination showed similar bone fill in experimental and control sites, whereas subjects receiving the rhPDGF-BB/IGF-I (150/150 μg/mL) combination showed statistically significant increased bone fill corresponding to a mean of 2.1-mm vertical gain (42% fill) compared with 0.8 mm (19% fill) for the controls. No serious local or systemic adverse effects attributable to treatments were observed. It is noteworthy that despite these encouraging observations, further studies on the rhPDGF-BB/IGF-1 combination have not been reported. Perhaps growth factor combinations for periodontal wound healing/regeneration may never be developed for clinical use because of the substantial, complex, and costly evaluation needed to meet regulatory demands.

DIFFERENTIATION FACTORS

Bone morphogenetic proteins (BMPs) form a unique family within the TGF-β superfamily of proteins and have essential roles in regulation of bone formation, maintenance, and repair. While BMPs are frequently referred to as growth factors, it is more precise to regard them as differentiation factors because BMPs play important roles in cell migration, proliferation, differentiation, and apoptosis, and are involved in morphogenesis and organogenesis in such diverse tissues and organs as kidney, eye, nervous system, lung, teeth, skin, and heart. More than 20 BMPs have been identified, and several trials have evaluated rhBMPs for tissue engineering.[57,58] BMP-2, -3 (osteogenin), -4, -6, -7 (also known as osteogenic protein-1 [OP-1]), -12 (also known as growth/differentiation factor-7 [GDF-7]), and -14 (also known as GDF-5, or cartilage derived morphogenetic protein-1 [CDMP-1]) have been evaluated for periodontal wound healing/regeneration (**Table 2**).

Bone Morphogenetic Protein–2

BMP-2 has been shown to induce bone formation in orthopedic, craniofacial, and oral settings.[59] Our studies, all using the critical-size supra-alveolar periodontal defect model, have evaluated the effect of BMP-2 on periodontal wound healing/ regeneration using a broad range of carrier matrices, dosages, and healing intervals, and adjunctive use of space-providing devices. Carrier technologies have included bioresorbable poly(D,L-lactide-co-glycolide) (PLGA) microparticles,[60] allogeneic demineralized bone matrix (DBM),[61] an absorbable bovine type I collagen sponge (ACS),[61–66] bovine bone mineral (Bio-Oss),[61] polylactic acid granules (Drilac),[61] a calcium phosphate cement (Ceredex),[59] and a hyaluronan sponge.[67] Nonresorbable[63,64] and biodegradable[67] macroporous space-providing devices have been used in some studies. RhBMP-2 dosages have ranged between 0.05 and 0.4 mg/ mL and healing intervals have ranged between 8 and 24[67] weeks. Application of rhBMP-2 induced significant bone formation, depending on the carrier system and the presence or absence of space-providing devices. Also, significant formation of cementum or a cementumlike substance on the root surface was induced. However, a functionally oriented PDL has not been observed. Rather, fibrovascular tissue occupies the PDL space after 4 to 8 weeks of healing. After 24 weeks, that tissue morphs into fatty marrow, bone, and root resorption/ankylosis.[67]

However, not all studies evaluating rhBMP-2 for periodontal wound healing/regeneration report root resorption/ankylosis. RhBMP-2 (0.4 mg/mL) in a sponge-type gelatin/polylactic acid polyglycolic acid copolymer carrier significantly increased bone, cementum, and PDL formation in mandibular horizontal circumferential defects in dogs by 12 weeks postsurgery.[68] Baboon three-wall intrabony periodontal defects implanted with rhBMP-2/ACS and rhBMP-2/α-BSM (a calcium phosphate cement) showed significantly greater regeneration than carrier controls at 16 weeks.[69] Surgical implantation of rhBMP-2/ACS into three-wall intrabony periodontal defects in dogs resulted in accelerated, enhanced bone formation without apparent enhanced cementum regeneration using 8- and 24-week healing intervals. Also, no root resorption/ankylosis was observed.[70] Attempts to control root resorption/ankylosis have included a polymer-coated gelatin sponge and spacer membrane using horizontal circumferential defects in dogs and a 12-week healing interval.[71] Although the device eliminated root resorption/ankylosis, it also reduced bone formation, which in itself may explain the effects on ankylosis.

Collectively, preclinical evaluations of BMP-2 for periodontal indications demonstrate significantly enhanced bone and cementum formation compared with controls, but not a functionally oriented PDL. The significance of this observation is unclear and it must be noted that formation of a periodontal attachment following application of rhBMP-2 has also been reported. These evaluations highlight the critical influence of the carrier technology on treatment outcomes. RhBMP-2 applications frequently result in root resorption/ankylosis. RhBMP-2–associated ankylosis appears to be associated with rapid bone formation and may not be a significant aberration in the absence of extensive bone regeneration in more limited periodontal defects. The possibility of resolution of ankylosis has also been suggested in association with BMP-2 application in periodontal defects.[86] However, it should be recognized that these are cross-sectional observations. Such observations may be merely incidental and the conclusions regarding ankylosis resolution should be considered speculative. Results from clinical trials evaluating rhBMP-2 for periodontal indications have not been reported.

Bone Morphogenetic Protein–3 (Osteogenin)

BMP-3 has been evaluated for periodontal wound healing/regeneration in nonhuman primates and in humans.[72,73] In a human biopsy case series, purified hBMP-3 was combined with demineralized freeze-dried bone or bovine tendon–derived collagen

Table 2
Effect of differentiation factors on periodontal wound healing/regeneration in preclinical models and pivotal clinical studies

Factor (Preclinical or Clinical)	Model; Platform	Dose; Carrier; Healing Interval	Major Observation	References
BMP-2 (preclinical)	Supra-alveolar; dog	0.05–0.4 mg/mL; PLGA, DBM, PLA, ACS, CP cement, HY sponge; 8, 24 wk	Significant bone and cementum formation, no PDL, root resorption/ankylosis	59–67
	Supra-alveolar; dog	0.4 mg/mL; gelatin/PLGA; 12 wk	Enhanced bone, cementum, PDL	68
	3-wall intrabony; nonhuman primate	0.4 mg/mL; ACS, α-BSM; 16 wk	Enhanced periodontal regeneration	69
	3-wall intrabony; dog	0.2 mg/mL; ACS; 8, 24 wk	Enhanced bone but not cementum formation	70
	Supra-alveolar; dog	0.1 mg/mL; gelatin sponge, spacer membrane; 12 wk	Spacer eliminated root resorption/ankylosis, but reduced bone formation	71
BMP-3/osteogenin (preclinical)	Class II furcation; nonhuman primate	250 µg/site; type I collagen; 8 wk	Enhanced PDL and bone formation	72
BMP-3; osteogenin (clinical)	Case series, 16 patients, intrabony defects; clinical and biopsies	200 µg/site; type I collagen; 6 mo	Enhanced periodontal regeneration	73
BMP-6 (preclinical)	Fenestration/rat	0, 1, 3, 10 µg/site; type I collagen; 4 wk	3 µg: greatest bone and cementum formation	74
BMP-7/OP-1 (preclinical)	Class II furcation; nonhuman primate	0, 100, 500 µg/g; type I collagen; 8 wk	Enhanced cementogenesis and PDL	75
	Class II furcation; nonhuman primate	0.5, 2.5 mg/g; type I collagen; 24 wk	Enhanced PDL and alveolar bone formation	76
	Class III furcation; dog	0.75, 2.5, 7.5 mg/g; type I collage; 8 wk	Enhanced periodontal regeneration	77
	Class II furcation; nonhuman primate; (rhBMP-2 vs rhOP-1)	100 µg/g; type I collagen; 8 wk	RhOP-1: enhanced cementogenesis; rhBMP-2: enhanced bone formation	78

BMP-12/GDF-7 (preclinical)	Supra-alveolar; dog (GDF-7 vs rhBMP-2)	GDF-7: 0.04, 0.1, 0.2 mg/mL; ACS; 8 wk. RhBMP-2: 0.2 mg/mL; ACS; 8 wk	GDF-7: PDL regeneration. RhBMP-2: no PDL formation	66
BMP-14/GDF-5 (preclinical)	1-wall intrabony; dog	20 μg/site; β-TCP; 8 wk	Enhanced bone and cementum formation, PDL	79
	1-wall intrabony; dog	1, 20, 100 μg/site; ACS; 8 wk	Enhanced bone and cementum formation, PDL	80
	Supra-alveolar; dog	500 μg/g β-TCP; PLGA; 8 wk	Enhanced cementum and bone formation, PDL	81
	Dehiscence; dog	93 μg/site; PLGA; 2, 4, 6, 8 wk	Accelerated bone regeneration	82
	1-wall intrabony; dog	RhGDF-5: 500 μg/g; β-TCP; 8 wk. RhPDGF: 0.3 mg/mL; β-TCP; 8 wk	RhGDF-5: enhanced bone and cementum formation over rhPDGF	83
BMP-14/GDF-5 (clinical)	Phase IIa randomized controlled trial, 20 patients, ≥4-mm intrabony defects; clinical and biopsies	500 μg rhGDF-5/g; β-TCP; 6 mo	Twice greater clinical attachment gain, favorable bone and periodontal regeneration	84,85

Abbreviations: ACS, absorbable collagen sponge; CP, calcium phosphate; DBM, demineralized bone matrix; HY, hyaluronan; PLA, polylactic acid; PLGA, poly(D,L-lactide-co-glycolide).

matrices and implanted into intrabony periodontal defects in teeth slated for extraction.[73] The histometric evaluation showed that BMP-3 significantly enhanced periodontal regeneration compared with carrier controls in submerged but not in nonsubmerged defect sites following a 6-month healing interval. This first indication that BMPs may stimulate periodontal wound healing/regeneration, was corroborated in a nonhuman primate model. A purified construct predominantly containing BMP-3 (but also BMP-2 and BMP-7) in collagen carrier was implanted into surgically created mandibular molar class II furcation defects in baboons.[72] Histologic evaluation following an 8-week healing interval showed significantly greater PDL and bone formation in sites receiving BMP-3 compared with carrier control. The newly formed PDL exhibited Sharpey fibers inserting into newly deposited cementoid and showing nascent foci of mineralization. Despite these promising observations, further evaluation of the use of BMP-3 for periodontal regeneration has not been published.

Bone Morphogenetic Protein–6

The published record on BMP-6 for periodontal wound healing/regeneration is limited. BMP-6 (0, 1, 3, and 10 μg) in a type I collagen sponge carrier was applied into periodontal fenestration defects in rats.[74] Control defects received carrier alone. Complete osseous healing occurred in BMP-6–treated animals following a 4-week healing interval. With the BMP-6 dose apparently affecting bone and cementum formation, the 3-μg group exhibited the greatest bone and cementum formation. Limited bone formation was observed in the control. These initial observations warrant additional evaluation of BMP-6 in discriminating large animal models before clinical evaluation.

Bone Morphogenetic Protein–7 (Osteogenic Protein–1)

BMP-7, more commonly known as osteogenic protein-1 (OP-1), has been evaluated for periodontal wound healing/regeneration using surgically induced mandibular molar class II furcation defects in baboons.[75] Defects implanted with rhOP-1 at 0, 100, and 500 μg/g bovine bone insoluble collagen matrix were subject to histometric analysis following an 8-week healing interval. Sites receiving rhOP-1 showed significant cementogenesis, including inserting Sharpey fibers, while limited regeneration was observed in controls. A similar study using a 24-week healing interval showed that rhOP-1 at 0.5 and 2.5 mg/g collagen matrix induced significantly greater PDL and alveolar bone formation compared with carrier control.[76] Improved outcomes may be due to increased OP-1 dosages and an extended healing interval allowing spatially correct morphogenesis of the periodontal tissues. Significantly enhanced periodontal regeneration following application of rhOP-1 (0.75, 2.5, 7.5 mg OP-1/g collagen) compared with carrier or sham-surgery controls was also shown using class III furcation defects in dogs and an 8-week healing interval.[77] While sites treated with OP-1 showed pronounced bone, cementum, and PDL formation, the rhOP-1 treatment did not prevent root resorption/ankylosis. In a separate study, an rhOP-1/rhBMP-2 construct was compared with individual application of rhOP-1 or rhBMP-2 at 100 μg/g collagen matrix in baboon furcation defects.[78] The histologic analysis following an 8-week healing interval showed substantial cementogenesis with scattered remnants of the collagen carrier in rhOP-1–treated specimens. RhBMP-2 induced greater amounts of bone compared with rhOP-1 or the rhOP-1/rhBMP-2 construct, while the combination protocol did not enhance alveolar bone or PDL formation over individual application of rhBMP-2 or rhOP-1. Collectively, these observations demonstrate beneficial effects of OP-1 as a candidate therapeutic agent for periodontal wound healing/regeneration. However, the possibility of root resorption/ankylosis must be further explored. Nevertheless, clinical trials evaluating this technology for periodontal indications have not yet been published.

Bone Morphogenetic Protein–12 (Growth and Differentiation Factor–7)

BMP-12, also known as growth and differentiation factor-7 (GDF-7), induces tendon and ligamentlike tissue in vivo.[87] The potential of GDF-7 to stimulate PDL formation was evaluated in the critical-size, supra-alveolar periodontal defect model in a pilot study format.[66] A functionally oriented PDL that approached the density of the native PDL and bridged the gap between newly formed cementum and alveolar bone was uniquely observed in sites receiving recombinant human GDF-7 (rhGDF-7)/ACS following the 8-week healing interval. This pilot study suggests that GDF-7 has a significant potential to support regeneration of the PDL. Nevertheless additional evaluations are necessary before clinical introduction.

Bone Morphogenetic Protein–14 (Growth and Differentiation Factor–5, Cartilage Derived Morphogenetic Protein–1)

BMP-14, generally recognized as GDF-5, plays crucial roles in skeletal, tendon, and ligament morphogenesis.[87] MRNA-encoding GDF-5 is expressed during odontogenesis and GDF-5 may play a role in the formation of alveolar bone and the PDL.[88–90] The effect of GDF-5 on periodontal wound healing/regeneration has been evaluated using an established canine defect model.[2] Surgically created bilateral, critical-size, mandibular, one-wall, intrabony periodontal defects were implanted with rhGDF-5 at 20 μg in a β-TCP carrier or at 1, 20, 100 μg in an ACS carrier.[79,80] Controls received the β-TCP biomaterial or ACS alone, or sham surgery. The rhGDF-5 groups exhibited significantly enhanced bone and cementum formation, including a functionally oriented PDL, over that observed in the controls following an 8-week healing interval. The rhGDF-5/β-TCP construct was the most successful treatment. Few, if any, adverse reactions were observed. Other studies evaluated injectable PLGA carriers for ease of use and minimally invasive protocols,[81] while still others evaluated moldable composite carriers for onlay indications.[82] A Food and Drug Administration–approved rhPDGF/β-TCP construct (GEM 21S) was used to establish a benchmark for the competitive value of the rhGDF-5/β-TCP candidate treatment for periodontal wound healing/regeneration. One-wall, intrabony periodontal defects received rhGDF-5/β-TCP and rhPDGF/β-TCP in contralateral jaw quadrants.[83] RhGDF-5/β-TCP promoted significantly greater (2–2.5×) bone and cementum formation compared with rhPDGF/β-TCP. These promising results warranted follow-up clinical investigations.

A phase IIa randomized, controlled, clinical and histologic pilot parallel group study in 20 patients was conducted to evaluate the effect of the rhGDF-5/β-TCP construct versus that following sham-surgery control in advanced intrabony periodontal defects on teeth planned for extraction.[84,85] The results following a 6-month healing interval suggest that rhGDF-5/β-TCP is safe; no significant adverse reactions were noted. Less gingival recession and almost two times greater clinical attachment gain were observed for the rhGDF-5/β-TCP–treated sites. The histologic evaluation suggests that rhGDF-5/β-TCP favorably affects bone formation, and may substantially support periodontal regeneration.

SUMMARY

Several growth and differentiation factors have shown potential as therapeutic agents to support periodontal wound healing/regeneration, although optimal dosage, release kinetics, and suitable delivery systems are still unknown. Experimental variables, including delivery systems, dose, and the common use of poorly characterized preclinical models make it difficult to discern the genuine efficacy of each of these factors. Only a few growth and differentiation factors have reached clinical evaluation. It appears that well-defined discriminating preclinical models followed by well-designed clinical trials are needed to further investigate the true potential of these and other candidate factors. Thus, current research is focused on finding relevant growth and differentiation factors, optimal dosages, and the best approaches for delivery to develop clinically meaningful therapies in patient-centered settings.

REFERENCES

1. American Academy of Periodontology. Glossary of periodontal terms. 3rd Edition 1992. Chicago (IL): American Academy of Periodontology.
2. Kim CS, Choi SH, Chai JK, et al. Periodontal repair in surgically created intrabony defects in dogs: influence of the number of bone walls on healing response. J Periodontol 2004;75:229–35.
3. Wikesjö UME, Kean CJC, Zimmerman GJ. Periodontal repair in dogs: supraalveolar defect models for evaluation of safety and efficacy of periodontal reconstructive therapy. J Periodontol 1994;65:1151–7.
4. Wang HL, Pappert TD, Castelli WA, et al. The effect of platelet-derived growth factor on the cellular response of the periodontium: an autoradiographic study on dogs. J Periodontol 1994;65:429–36.
5. Cho MI, Lin WL, Genco RJ. Platelet-derived growth factor-modulated guided tissue regenerative therapy. J Periodontol 1995;66:522–30.
6. Park JB, Matsuura M, Han KY, et al. Periodontal regeneration in class III furcation defects of beagle dogs using guided tissue regenerative therapy with platelet-derived growth factor. J Periodontol 1995;66:462–77.
7. Giannobile WV, Hernandez RA, Finkelman RD, et al. Comparative effects of platelet-derived growth factor-BB and insulin-like growth factor-I, individually and in combination, on periodontal regeneration in macaca fascicularis. J Periodont Res 1996;31:301–12.
8. Nevins M, Giannobile WV, McGuire MK, et al. Platelet-derived growth factor stimulates bone fill and rate of attachment level gain: results of a large multicenter randomized controlled trial. J Periodontol 2005;76:2205–15.
9. Ridgway H, Mellonig JT, Cochran DL. Human histologic and clinical evaluation of recombinant human platelet-derived growth factor and beta-tricalcium phosphate for the treatment of periodontal intraosseous defects. Int J Periodontics Restorative Dent 2008;28:171–9.
10. Murakami S, Takayama S, Ikezawa K, et al. Regeneration of periodontal tissues by basic fibroblast growth factor. J Periodont Res 1999;34:425–30.
11. Murakami S, Takayama S, Kitamura M, et al. Recombinant human basic fibroblast growth factor (bFGF) stimulates periodontal regeneration in class II furcation defects created in beagle dogs. J Periodont Res 2003;38:97–103.
12. Takayama S, Murakami S, Shimabukuro Y, et al. Periodontal regeneration by FGF-2 (bFGF) in primate models. J Dent Res 2001;80:2075–9.
13. Rossa C Jr, Marcantonio E Jr, Cirelli JA, et al. Regeneration of class III furcation defects with basic fibroblast growth factor (b-FGF) associated with GTR. A descriptive and histometric study in dogs. J Periodontol 2000;71:775–84.
14. Sato Y, Kikuchi M, Ohata N, et al. Enhanced cementum formation in experimentally induced cementum defects of the root surface with the application of

recombinant basic fibroblast growth factor in collagen gel in vivo. J Periodontol 2004;75:243–8.

15. Kitamura M, Nakashima K, Kowashi Y, et al. Periodontal tissue regeneration using fibroblast growth factor-2: randomized controlled phase II clinical trial. PLoS ONE 2008;3:e2611.

16. Mohammed S, Pack AR, Kardos TB. The effect of transforming growth factor beta one (TGF-ß₁) on wound healing, with or without barrier membranes, in a class II furcation defect in sheep. J Periodont Res 1998;33:335–44.

17. Wikesjö UME, Razi SS, Sigurdsson TJ, et al. Periodontal repair in dogs: effect of recombinant human transforming growth factor-ß₁ on guided tissue regeneration. J Clin Periodontol 1998;25:475–81.

18. Tatakis DN, Wikesjö UME, Razi SS, et al. Periodontal repair in dogs: effect of transforming growth factor-ß₁ on alveolar bone and cementum regeneration. J Clin Periodontol 2000;27:698–704.

19. Wikesjö UME, Lim WH, Razi SS, et al. Periodontal repair in dogs: a bioabsorbable calcium carbonate coral implant enhances space provision for alveolar bone regeneration in conjunction with guided tissue regeneration. J Periodontol 2003;74:957–64.

20. Koo KT, Susin C, Wikesjö UME, et al. Transforming growth factor-ß₁ accelerates resorption of a calcium carbonate biomaterial in periodontal defects. J Periodontol 2007;78:723–9.

21. Moon IS, Chai JK, Cho KS, et al. Effects of polyglactin mesh combined with resorbable calcium carbonate or replamineform hydroxyapatite on periodontal repair in dogs. J Clin Periodontol 1996;23:945–51.

22. Teare JA, Ramoshebi LN, Ripamonti U. Periodontal tissue regeneration by recombinant human transforming growth factor-beta 3 in *Papio ursinus*. J Periodont Res 2008;43:1–8.

23. Lynch SE, de Castilla GR, Williams RC, et al. The effects of short-term application of a combination of platelet-derived and insulin-like growth factors on periodontal wound healing. J Periodontol 1991;62:458–67.

24. Lynch SE, Williams RC, Polson AM, et al. A combination of platelet-derived and insulin-like growth factors enhances periodontal regeneration. J Clin Periodontol 1989;16:545–8.

25. Howell TH, Fiorellini JP, Paquette DW, et al. A phase I/II clinical trial to evaluate a combination of recombinant human platelet-derived growth factor-BB and recombinant human insulin-like growth factor-I in patients with periodontal disease. J Periodontol 1997;68:1186–93.

26. Hollinger JO, Hart CE, Hirsch SN, et al. Recombinant human platelet-derived growth factor: biology and clinical applications. J Bone Joint Surg Am 2008;90: 48–54.

27. Bergsten E, Uutela M, Li X, et al. PDGF-D is a specific, protease-activated ligand for the PDGF beta-receptor. Nat Cell Biol 2001;3:512–6.

28. Uutela M, Lauren J, Bergsten E, et al. Chromosomal location, exon structure, and vascular expression patterns of the human PDGFC and PDGFC genes. Circulation 2001;103:2242–7.

29. Green RJ, Usui ML, Hart CE, et al. Immunolocalization of platelet-derived growth factor A and B chains and PDGF-alpha and beta receptors in human gingival wounds. J Periodont Res 1997;32:209–14.

30. Dennison DK, Vallone DR, Pinero GJ, et al. Differential effect of TGF-beta 1 and PDGF on proliferation of periodontal ligament cells and gingival fibroblasts. J Periodontol 1994;65:641–8.

31. Matsuda N, Lin WL, Kumar NM, et al. Mitogenic, chemotactic, and synthetic responses of rat periodontal ligament fibroblastic cells to polypeptide growth factors in vitro. J Periodontol 1992;63:515–25.
32. Oates TW, Rouse CA, Cochran DL. Mitogenic effects of growth factors on human periodontal ligament cells in vitro. J Periodontol 1993;64:142–8.
33. Ojima Y, Mizuno M, Kuboki Y, et al. In vitro effect of platelet-derived growth factor-BB on collagen synthesis and proliferation of human periodontal ligament cells. Oral Dis 2003;9:144–51.
34. Boyan LA, Bhargava G, Nishimura F, et al. Mitogenic and chemotactic responses of human periodontal ligament cells to the different isoforms of platelet-derived growth factor. J Dent Res 1994;73:1593–600.
35. Zaman KU, Sugaya T, Kato H. Effect of recombinant human platelet-derived growth factor-BB and bone morphogenetic protein-2 application to demineralized dentin on early periodontal ligament cell response. J Periodont Res 1999;34:244–50.
36. Giannobile WV, Lee CS, Tomala MP, et al. Platelet-derived growth factor (PDGF) gene delivery for application in periodontal tissue engineering. J Periodontol 2001;72:815–23.
37. Saygin NE, Tokiyasu Y, Giannobile WV, et al. Growth factors regulate expression of mineral associated genes in cementoblasts. J Periodontol 2000;71:1591–600.
38. Butler AA, Le Roith D. Minireview: tissue-specific versus generalized gene argeting of the igf1 and igf1r genes and their roles in insulin-like growth factor physiology. Endocrinology 2001;142:1685–8.
39. Butler AA, Yakar S, Gewolb IH, et al. Insulin-like growth factor-I receptor signal transduction: at the interface between physiology and cell biology. Comp Biochem Physiol B Biochem Mol Biol 1998;121:19–26.
40. Baylink DJ, Finkelman RD, Mohan S. Growth factors to stimulate bone formation. J Bone Miner Res 1993;8(Suppl 2):S565–72.
41. Canalis E. Insulin-like growth factors and osteoporosis. Bone 1997;21:215–6.
42. Hock JM, Centrella M, Canalis E. Insulin-like growth factor I has independent effects on bone matrix formation and cell replication. Endocrinology 1988;122:254–60.
43. Schoenle E, Zapf J, Humbel RE, et al. Insulin-like growth factor I stimulates growth in hypophysectomized rats. Nature 1982;296:252–3.
44. Mochizuki H, Hakeda Y, Wakatsuki N, et al. Insulin-like growth factor-I supports formation and activation of osteoclasts. Endocrinology 1992;131:1075–80.
45. Nishimura F, Terranova VP. Comparative study of the chemotactic responses of periodontal ligament cells and gingival fibroblasts to polypeptide growth factors. J Dent Res 1996;75:986–92.
46. Palioto DB, Coletta RD, Graner E, et al. The influence of enamel matrix derivative associated with insulin-like growth factor-I on periodontal ligament fibroblasts. J Periodontol 2004;75:498–504.
47. Lynch SE, Williams RC, Polson AM, et al. Effect of insulin-like growth factor-I on periodontal regeneration. J Dent Res 1989;68:394.
48. Globus RK, Plouet J, Gospodarowicz D. Cultured bovine bone cells synthesize basic fibroblast growth factor and store it in their extracellular matrix. Endocrinology 1989;124:1539–47.
49. Hauschka PV, Mavrakos AE, Iafrati MD, et al. Growth factors in bone matrix. Isolation of multiple types by affinity chromatography on heparin-sepharose. J Biol Chem 1986;261:12665–74.
50. de Moerlooze L, Dickson C. Skeletal disorders associated with fibroblast growth factor receptor mutations. Curr Opin Genet Dev 1997;7:378–85.

51. Kress W, Collmann H, Büsse M, et al. Clustering of FGFR2 gene mutations in patients with Pfeiffer and Crouzon syndromes (FGFR2-associated craniosynostoses). Cytogenet Cell Genet 2000;91:134–7.
52. Kato T, Kawaguchi H, Hanada K, et al. Single local injection of recombinant fibroblast growth factor-2 stimulates healing of segmental bone defects in rabbits. J Orthop Res 1998;16:654–9.
53. Parkar MH, Kuru L, Giouzeli M, et al. Expression of growth-factor receptors in normal and regenerating human periodontal cells. Arch Oral Biol 2001;46: 275–84.
54. Sant'Ana AC, Marques MM, Barroso TE, et al. Effects of TGF-β$_1$, PDGF-BB, and IGF-1 on the rate of proliferation and adhesion of a periodontal ligament cell lineage in vitro. J Periodontol 2007;78:2007–17.
55. Giannobile WV, Whitson SW, Lynch SE. Non-coordinate control of bone formation displayed by growth factor combinations with IGF-I. J Dent Res 1997;76: 1569–78.
56. Lynch SE, Colvin RB, Antoniades HN. Growth factors in wound healing. Single and synergistic effects on partial thickness porcine skin wounds. J Clin Invest 1989;84:640–6.
57. Reddi AH. Bone morphogenetic proteins: from basic science to clinical applications. J Bone Joint Surg Am 2001;83-A:S1–6.
58. Reddi AH. Role of morphogenetic proteins in skeletal tissue engineering and regeneration. Nat Biotechnol 1998;16:247–52.
59. Sorensen RG, Wikesjö UME, Kinoshita A, et al. Periodontal repair in dogs: evaluation of a bioresorbable calcium phosphate cement (Ceredex) as a carrier for rhBMP-2. J Clin Periodontol 2004;31:796–804.
60. Sigurdsson TJ, Lee MB, Kubota K, et al. Periodontal repair in dogs: recombinant human bone morphogenetic protein-2 significantly enhances periodontal regeneration. J Periodontol 1995;66:131–8.
61. Sigurdsson TJ, Nygaard L, Tatakis DN, et al. Periodontal repair in dogs: evaluation of rhBMP-2 carriers. Int J Periodontics Restorative Dent 1996;16:524–37.
62. Selvig KA, Sorensen RG, Wozney JM, et al. Bone repair following recombinant human bone morphogenetic protein-2 stimulated periodontal regeneration. J Periodontol 2002;73:1020–9.
63. Wikesjö UME, Xiropaidis AV, Thomson RC, et al. Periodontal repair in dogs: RhBMP-2 significantly enhances bone formation under provisions for guided tissue regeneration. J Clin Periodontol 2003;30:705–14.
64. Wikesjö UME, Xiropaidis AV, Thomson RC, et al. Periodontal repair in dogs: Space-providing ePTFE devices increase rhBMP-2/ACS-induced bone formation. J Clin Periodontol 2003;30:715–25.
65. Wikesjö UME, Guglielmoni P, Promsudthi A, et al. Periodontal repair in dogs: effect of rhBMP-2 concentration on regeneration of alveolar bone and periodontal attachment. J Clin Periodontol 1999;26:392–400.
66. Wikesjö UME, Sorensen RG, Kinoshita A, et al. Periodontal repair in dogs: effect of recombinant human bone morphogenetic protein-12 (rhBMP-12) on regeneration of alveolar bone and periodontal attachment. J Clin Periodontol 2004;31: 662–70.
67. Wikesjö UME, Lim WH, Thomson RC, et al. Periodontal repair in dogs: evaluation of a bioabsorbable space-providing macroporous membrane with recombinant human bone morphogenetic protein-2. J Periodontol 2003;74:635–47.
68. Kinoshita A, Oda S, Takahashi K, et al. Periodontal regeneration by application of recombinant human bone morphogenetic protein-2 to horizontal circumferential

defects created by experimental periodontitis in beagle dogs. J Periodontol 1997;68:103–9.

69. Blumenthal NM, Koh-Kunst G, Alves ME, et al. Effect of surgical implantation of recombinant human bone morphogenetic protein-2 in a bioabsorbable collagen sponge or calcium phosphate putty carrier in intrabony periodontal defects in the baboon. J Periodontol 2002;73:1494–506.

70. Choi SH, Kim CK, Cho KS, et al. Effect of recombinant human bone morphogenetic protein-2/absorbable collagen sponge (rhBMP-2/ACS) on healing in 3-wall intrabony defects in dogs. J Periodontol 2002;73:63–72.

71. Saito E, Saito A, Kawanami M. Favorable healing following space creation in rhBMP-2-induced periodontal regeneration of horizontal circumferential defects in dogs with experimental periodontitis. J Periodontol 2003;74:1808–15.

72. Ripamonti U, Heliotis M, van den Heever B, et al. Bone morphogenetic proteins induce periodontal regeneration in the baboon (*Papio ursinus*). J Periodont Res 1994;29:439–45.

73. Bowers G, Felton F, Middleton C, et al. Histologic comparison of regeneration in human intrabony defects when osteogenin is combined with demineralized freeze-dried bone allograft and with purified bovine collagen. J Periodontol 1991;62:690–702.

74. Huang KK, Shen C, Chiang CY, et al. Effects of bone morphogenetic protein-6 on periodontal wound healing in a fenestration defect of rats. J Periodont Res 2005; 40:1–10.

75. Ripamonti U, Heliotis M, Rueger DC, et al. Induction of cementogenesis by recombinant human osteogenic protein-1 (hOP-1/BMP-7) in the baboon (*Papio ursinus*). Arch Oral Biol 1996;41:121–6.

76. Ripamonti U, Crooks J, Teare J, et al. Periodontal tissue regeneration by recombinant human osteogenic protein-1 in periodontally-induced furcation defects of the primate *Papio ursinus*. S Afr J Sci 2002;98:361–8.

77. Giannobile WV, Ryan S, Shih MS, et al. Recombinant human osteogenic protein-1 (OP-1) stimulates periodontal wound healing in class III furcation defects. J Periodontol 1998;69:129–37.

78. Ripamonti U, Crooks J, Petit JC, et al. Periodontal tissue regeneration by combined applications of recombinant human osteogenic protein-1 and bone morphogenetic protein-2. A pilot study in Chacma baboons (*Papio ursinus*). Eur J Oral Sci 2001;109:241–8.

79. Lee JS, Wikesjö UM, Kim YT, et al. rhGDF-5 in a ß-tricalcium phosphate carrier significantly supports periodontal regeneration. J Dent Res 2009;88, (Special Issue A) IADR-abstract 2185.

80. Kim TG, Wikesjö UM, Cho KS, et al. Periodontal regeneration following implantation of rhGDF-5 in a collagen carrier. J Dent Res 2009;88, (Special Issue A) IADR-abstract 2193.

81. Kwon D, Bisch F, Herold R, et al. Effect of rhGDF-5 in a novel carrier on periodontal regeneration. J Dent Res 2009;88. (Special Issue A) IADR-abstract 1593.

82. Bennett W, Kwon D, Rodriguez NA, et al. An injectable rhGDF-5 composite for minimally invasive periodontal regenerative procedures. J Dent Res 2009;88, (Special Issue A) IADR-abstract 2192.

83. Kwon HR, Wikesjö UM, Jung UW, et al. Periodontal regeneration following implantation of rhGDF-5 vs. rhPDGF in dogs. J Dent Res 2009;88, (Special Issue A) IADR-abstract 1711.

84. Stavropoulos A, Sculean A, Wikesjö UM, et al. A phase IIA randomized, controlled, clinical & histological pilot study evaluating rhGDF-5/ß-TCP for

periodontal regeneration. Histological results. J Clin Periodontol 2009;36, (Special Issue s9) Abstracts of Europerio 6 Ref no: EUABS064243.

85. Windisch P, Stavropoulos A, Sculean A, et al. A phase IIA randomized, controlled, clinical and histological pilot study evaluating rhGDF-5/β-TCP for periodontal regeneration. Clinical results. J Clin Periodontol 2009;36, (Special Issues 9) Abstracts of Europerio 6 Ref no: EUABS065945.

86. Takahashi D, Odajima T, Morita M, et al. Formation and resolution of ankylosis under application of recombinant human bone morphogenetic protein-2 (rhBMP-2) to class III furcation defects in cats. J Periodont Res 2005;40:299–305.

87. Wolfman NM, Hattersley G, Cox K, et al. Ectopic induction of tendon and ligament in rats by growth and differentiation factors 5, 6, and 7, members of the TGF-beta gene family. J Clin Invest 1997;100:321–30.

88. Nakamura T, Yamamoto M, Tamura M, et al. Effects of growth/differentiation factor-5 on human periodontal ligament cells. J Periodont Res 2003;38:597–605.

89. Sena K, Morotome Y, Baba O, et al. Gene expression of growth differentiation factors in the developing periodontium of rat molars. J Dent Res 2003;82:166–71.

90. Morotome Y, Goseki-Sone M, Ishikawa I, et al. Gene expression of growth and differentiation factors-5, -6, and -7 in developing bovine tooth at the root forming stage. Biochem Biophys Res Commun 1998;244:85–90.

Dental Implants in the Periodontal Patient

Gary Greenstein, DDS, MS[a,b],*, John Cavallaro Jr, DDS[a,b],
Dennis Tarnow, DDS[a,b]

KEYWORDS

- Dental implants • Periodontitis • Risk factors

The principal reason for providing periodontal therapy is to achieve periodontal health and retain the dentition. This objective includes restitution of form and function, esthetics, and avoidance of further periodontal disease progression.[1] Although not mandatory to sustain life, many people prefer to have a full or functioning dentition. Replacement of lost teeth with conventional prostheses on natural teeth or with dental implants is desirable. In this regard, osseointegration of dental implants is a predictable treatment modality and an integral aspect of treatment planning in the periodontal patient who has or is expected to lose teeth.[2,3] Patients with a history of periodontitis, however, represent a unique group of individuals who previously succumbed to a bacterial challenge. Therefore, it was deemed important to address the management and survival rate of implants in these patients. Systematic reviews often are cited in this article, because they provide a high level of evidence and facilitate reviewing a vast amount of information in a succinct manner.

MAJOR CAUSES OF TOOTH LOSS IN PATIENTS

It has been questioned whether dental caries or periodontal diseases are the main cause of tooth loss. Several investigations have indicated the main reason for tooth extraction in all age groups is caries[4,5]; however, others suggest it is periodontal diseases.[2,6–8] An apparent interpretation of their findings is that caries causes tooth loss in more patients, but periodontal diseases are responsible for more teeth being removed in individual patients.[8,9] In addition, periodontitis is the principal reason for edentulism in individuals vulnerable to periodontal diseases.[9–11] Because more teeth are lost due to periodontal disease than any other oral affliction, the issue as to the

[a] Department of Periodontology & Implant Dentistry, New York University College of Dentistry, 900 West Main Street, Freehold, NJ 07728, USA
[b] Private Practice
* Corresponding author. Department of Periodontology & Implant Dentistry, New York University College of Dentistry, 900 West Main Street, Freehold, NJ 07728, USA.
E-mail address: ggperio@aol.com (G. Greenstein).

Dent Clin N Am 54 (2010) 113–128
doi:10.1016/j.cden.2009.08.008
0011-8532/09/$ – see front matter © 2010 Elsevier Inc. All rights reserved.

success of placing dental implants in patients with a history of periodontitis is an important treatment planning consideration.

ETIOLOGIC AGENTS OF PERIODONTITIS AND PERI-IMPLANTITIS

Bacteria are the main etiologic agents that induce periodontitis and peri-implantitis[12]; therefore, knowledge concerning the main pathogens is important for understanding the linkage between retention of implants and a patient's history of periodontitis. Within the human oral cavity, hundreds of species of bacteria have been identified.[13] In individuals with chronic periodontitis, it has been reported that the predominant bacterial species are gram-negative anaerobes; however, other microorganisms may be present. The main pathogens identified were *Porphyromonas gingivalis, Prevotella intermedia, Actinobacillus actinomycetemcomitans (Aggregatibacter actinomycetemcomitans), Bacteroides forsythus (Tannerella forsythensis),* and *Treponema.*[13] Numerous studies have indicated the composition of the microflora associated with periodontitis and peri-implantitis (bleeding and bone loss around an implant) are similar.[14–18] Furthermore, when Shibli and colleagues[19] compared the microflora around implants that manifested peri-implantitis and those that were healthy, it was noted that the same types of bacteria were present around diseased and healthy implants; but an increased quantity of bacteria was found at diseased sites.

With respect to the rate that bacteria from a tooth colonize an implant, Quirynen and colleagues[20] reported that initial subgingival colonization of implants with bacteria associated with periodontitis can occur within 2 weeks in partially edentate patients. On the other hand, in completely edentate individuals, Danser and colleagues[21] noted that the main reservoir of colonization for dental implants in edentulous patients was oral mucous membranes. After all teeth were removed due to periodontitis, they found that bacteria harbored by individuals with dental implants were species usually associated with a healthy periodontium or gingivitis. It was suggested that extraction of natural teeth resulted in elimination of two potential pathogens, *A actinomycetemcomitans and P gingivalis.* In contrast to these findings, however, others[22,23] indicated that implants placed into edentate individuals experienced re-emergence of bacterial pathogens by 6 months with an almost identical spectrum of pathogens, including *P gingivalis, T forsythensis,* and other pathogenic bacteria that were present before the teeth were extracted.

In summary, the finding that bacteria associated with implant health and disease are similar is not surprising, because most microbes located in the oral cavity are considered indigenous organisms.[24,25] Furthermore, it appears that teeth and other reservoirs of bacteria (mucous membranes, saliva, pharynx) in edentate patients have the potential to be a source of bacterial reinfection once implants are placed. This underscores the need to initiate periodontal therapy in patients with periodontitis before placing dental implants to reduce the level of potential pathogens, thereby inhibiting them from colonizing the implants and initiating peri-implantitis.

SURVIVAL OF IMPLANTS IN PATIENTS WITH A HISTORY OF PERIODONTITIS

Individuals who were fully or partially edentate were successfully rehabilitated using osseointegrated dental implants to support fixed prostheses.[26–29] The question remains as to whether these individual are at greater risk of developing peri-implantitis than patients who have not previously had periodontal diseases, and if they are, how great are the risks and what can be done to enhance successful therapy with implants.

Partially Edentulous Patients

Karoussis and colleagues[26] conducted a systematic review of the literature with respect to the success/survival rates of dental implants placed in patients with a history of periodontis who were partially dentate. Studies were assessed in two categories: short term (< 5 years) and long term (> 5 years) after osseointegrated implants were placed in periodontally compromised partially edentulous patients. Based upon 15 prospective investigations (seven short- and 8 long-term studies), the authors made the following observations. They found no statistically significant differences in the survival rates between the short- and long-term studies. However, when patients with a history of periodontitis were compared with individuals who were periodontally healthy, it was reported that patients with a history of periodontitis manifested significantly greater probing depths, more peri-implant marginal bone loss, and a higher incidence of peri-implantitis. It was concluded that implant survival rate was acceptable in individuals with a history of periodontitis who were in a maintenance program.

Fully Edentulous Patients

Several studies addressed the 15- to 20-year survival rates of implants placed in patients who were fully edentulous: For example, Astrand and colleagues[27] found a 99.2% survival rate for implants; Adell and colleagues[28] reported implant retention in the maxilla and mandible was 78% and 86%, respectively, and Jemt and Johansson[29] reported that the implant survival rate was 90.9%. It can be surmised that the long-term survival rates with implants seem satisfactory in edentate patients. It should be recognized, however, that these clinical trials did not specify that the involved patients had a history of periodontitis, which may affect the long-term survival rate.

Patients with a History of Aggressive Periodontitis

To clarify the success rate of implants in patients with a history of aggressive periodontitis (ie, juvenile and rapidly progressive periodontitis), Al-Zahrani[30] conducted a systematic review, which included nine articles, four of which were case reports. These publications demonstrated there was good short-term survival of implants placed in patients treated for aggressive periodontitis that subsequently were periodontally maintained. The data indicated, however, that bone loss occurred around implants in patients with a history of aggressive periodontitis more often than around implants in patients with history of chronic periodontitis or periodontally healthy individuals. In addition, the author made several comments that should be underscored to interpret these findings:

Periodontal diseases should be controlled before placement of implants.
Individuals with aggressive periodontitis may be susceptible to additional periods of disease progression. At present, however, no recommendations can be made to define a time period that should elapse before initiating implant therapy.
There are a limited number of studies addressing the survival rate in patients with aggressive periodontitis.
It is unknown what effect retention of questionable teeth in these patients will have on the success rate of implants in individuals who had aggressive periodontitis.

Implant Placement in Sites Augmented with Guided Bone Regeneration

Because patients with a history of periodontitis often require guided bone regeneration (GBR) procedures (bone graft with a barrier) to restore bone before implant placement, it was considered important to address survival of implants in grafted bone.

A recent systematic review (11 studies included) by Hammerle and colleagues[31] compared survival of implants in regenerated bone attained with GBR with survival of implants placed into native bone. The cumulative survival rates for implants in regenerated bone varied from 79.4% to 100% after 5 years of function. The authors concluded that there were no significant differences found in the controlled clinical trials with respect to survival rates between implants placed in regenerated bone compared with implants inserted in native bone. It should be recognized, however, that this review did not specifically look at patients with a history of periodontitis, which may affect the implant survival rate.

Implants in Sinus Augmented Bone

Several investigations specifically assessed the survival rate of implants placed into sinus grafts in patients who were periodontally compromised.[32,33] Ellegaard and colleagues monitored 24 patients for 36 to 42 months[32] and 68 patients for 10 years.[33] Both studies concurred that implants may be inserted into a sinus augmented with bone in periodontally compromised patients with the same success as implants placed in individuals without a history of periodontitis.

DIAGNOSTIC PARAMETERS TO ASSESS DENTAL IMPLANTS

The tissues that surround teeth and implants respond in a similar manner to a bacterial challenge. Peri-implant diseases consist of two entities: peri-implant mucositis that is similar to gingivitis, and peri-implantitis, which is comparable to periodontitis.[34] Mucositis denotes that there is inflammation of the tissue around an implant without any signs of bone loss. In contrast, peri-implantitis connotes mucosal inflammation and bone loss. There are a few parameters that can be used to diagnose peri-implant diseases.

Probing Depth

Deeper than usual probing depths around an implant may not indicate the presence of peri-implantitis, because an implant placed at various depths subgingivally can result in a deep sulcus.[35] Contributing to this finding is the fact that connective tissue fibers adhere to, but are not attached to an implant as they are to teeth; therefore, they do not impede probe tip penetration. Nevertheless, increasing probing depth over time is associated with loss of bone around an implant.[36] In health, the probe will penetrate to the apical extent of the epithelium, and the junctional epithelium heals within 5 days.[37] In peri-implantitis lesions, the probe will penetrate into the connective tissue. Stable probing depths in the absence of recession reflect stability of the tissues adjacent to the implant. In summary, it is prudent to probe around dental implants to assess periodontal peri-implant health during periodic examinations.[38]

Bleeding Upon Probing

Healthy implant sites manifest an absence of bleeding, whereas sites with mucositis or peri-implantitis demonstrate bleeding upon probing 67% and 91% of the time, respectively.[39] Most importantly, it has been reported that an absence of bleeding is an indicator for a stable peri-implant condition with respect to future attachment loss.[40]

Radiographs

Radiographs are a valuable aid in diagnosing loss of osseous support around an implant. Assessment of bone loss from the osseous crest to a fixed reference point (eg, osseous crest to implant–abutment connection) can be recorded; however, limitations of radiographs should be noted. For example, panoramic films have distortion of about 23%.[41] Furthermore, in general, radiographs underestimate bone loss, because a substantial amount of the buccal or lingual plate of bone needs to be demineralized before it seen radiographically. Additionally, there is an inability to differentiate between defects in the buccal or lingual plate of bone.[42] In contrast, computed tomography (CT) and cone beam volume imaging have provided accurate three-dimensional imaging of bone surrounding dental implants.[43,44]

Biochemical and Other Markers of Disease

There are no biochemical markers from the peri-implant crevicular fluid or microbiological tests that are good predictors for future disease progression around dental implants.[38] Mobility is not a useful clinical parameter to monitor implants, because its presence denotes a failed implant that needs to be removed.[38] On the other hand, suppuration reflects an infection, but its presence may or may not denote the presence of ongoing bone loss.[45]

RISK INDICATORS FOR PERI-IMPLANTITIS

Several risk indicators for peri-implantitis identified in cross-sectional and retrospective studies were investigated. These indicators, however, are not necessarily true risk factors (delineate a cause and effect relationship), which can be identified only by prospective clinical trials.

History of Periodontis

Heitz-Mayfield[38] assessed four systematic reviews that addressed the history of periodontitis as a risk factor for peri-implantitis. Despite variations in clinical trials with respect to their design and maintenance schedules, it was concluded that patients with a history of periodontitis are at greater risk for peri-implantitis than individuals who never have had periodontitis.

Diabetes

Only one investigation evaluated the relationship between peri-implantitis and diabetes. Ferreira and colleagues[46] concluded that poor metabolic control in subjects with diabetes was associated with peri-implantitis (odds ratio was 1:9).

Genetics

Cytokine gene polymorphisms may alter the host response to a bacterial challenge and affect susceptibility to peri-implantitis. A recent systematic review by Huynh-Ba and colleagues[47] found that there is not enough evidence to support an association between the interleukin (IL)-1 genotype status and peri-implantitis. Therefore, at present, genetic testing for the evaluation of the risk of peri-implantitis cannot be suggested as a standard of care.

Smoking

A systematic review (included six studies) by Strietzel and colleagues[48] noted that there was a significant increase in marginal bone loss around implants in smokers compared with nonsmokers. It was concluded that smokers are at increased risk of biologic complications (eg, peri-implantitis and reduced implant survival rate) compared with nonsmokers.

Oral Hygiene

Two investigations indicated that poor oral hygiene was a risk indicator for peri-implantitis. Ferreira and colleagues[46] noted that individuals with very poor oral hygiene had an increased odds ratio (14:3) of experiencing peri-implantitis compared with patients with good oral hygiene. Similarly, Linquist[49] reported that after 10 years, smokers with poor oral hygiene (plaque accumulation was monitored) had three times greater marginal bone loss than nonsmokers.

Absence of Keratinized Tissue

The role of keratinized gingiva in maintaining dental implants is a controversial issue. Based on long-term implant success and survival studies, there appears to be little or no difference in the survival rate for implants surrounded by oral mucosa or keratinized tissue.[50]

One paper, however, indicated that hydroxy apatite (HA)-coated implants had a higher survival rate when keratinized tissue was present.[51] With respect to tissue inflammation, recession, and bone loss, there is conflicting information in the literature. When there was a dearth of keratinized gingiva, several investigators reported there was a statistically significant increased amount of inflammation,[52] whereas others indicated the amount of inflammation was not increased when there was a lack of keratinized gingiva.[45,53,54] Some researchers found that the absence of keratinized gingiva was associated with a statistically significant increased amount of recession **(Fig. 1)**,[53,55] but this finding conflicted with the data of others.[56,57] Similarly, several studies concluded that the absence of keratinized gingiva was[51,53] or was not[45,58] associated with a statistically significant additional bone loss. A possible explanation for these contradictions is that with good oral hygiene, peri-implant soft tissue health can be maintained irrespective of the amount of keratinized gingival tissue surrounding implant/restoration present; however, if there is less than good oral hygiene, it may be advantageous to have keratinized gingiva.[50] In conclusion, despite a lack of data, some authors suggest that there may be situations when soft tissue augmentation at implant sites may need to be considered (eg, depending upon the site, dental history of the patient).[56] These recommendations to date, however, have no scientific basis.

Implant Surfaces

It should be noted that there are three types of surface roughness (Sa) on implants (minimally rough, Sa = 0.5 μm also referred to as machined implants, smooth, turned), moderately rough, Sa equal to 1 to 2 μm (eg, Osseotite [3i Implant Innovations, FL, USA], SLA [Straumann Company, MA, USA], TiUnite [Nobel Biocare, CA, USA]) and

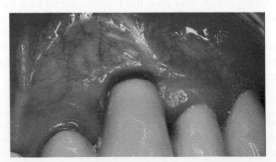

Fig. 1. At site #11, there is no attached keratinized gingiva. Despite the appearance of being healthy, there has been recession within the first year of the crown's placement.

rough, Sa greater than 2μm, (eg, plasma-sprayed and HA-coated implants)[59] and that with increasing roughness, implant surfaces attract and retain more bacteria.[60] There is limited and conflicting information, however, with respect to the impact of implant surface topography as a risk factor for peri-implantitis. In a dog model, investigators[61,62] noted that the progression of peri-implantitis, if left untreated, is greater around implants with a moderately rough surface than those with a polished surface. In humans, Astrand and colleagues[63] also found that rough-surfaced implants had a higher incidence of peri-implantitis than smooth (turned) surfaces, whereas, Wennstrom and colleagues[64] reported similar bone level changes for turned and relatively rough surface implants. Albouy and colleagues[65] compared the amount of induced disease progression (dog model) with respect to four different surfaces (turned, Tio-Blast [Astra Tech Inc, MA, USA], sandblasted acid-etched, and TiUnite). They reported that disease progression was most pronounced at implants with a TiUnite surface. In summary, at present, there is insufficient information in people to make a definitive determination as to whether the surface characteristic of the implant predisposes a patient to peri-implantitis.

PREVENTION, PREVALENCE, AND THERAPY FOR PATIENTS WITH PERI-IMPLANTITIS
Prevention of Peri-implantitis: Periodontal Supportive Therapy

It is appropriate that clinicians maintain a recall system for patients who receive implants in order to monitor them and provide supportive periodontal therapy (SPT).[66] In this regard, Quirynen and colleagues[66] reviewed 16 studies and concluded that periodontally compromised patients can be maintained successfully with moderately rough implants if they are provided SPT. With respect to the time interval between SPT visits, numerous investigations indicated that a 3-month interval is adequate for most periodontal patients[67]; but some patients need more or less frequent visits.

Prevalence of Peri-Implantitis

Zitzmann and Berglundh[35] conducted a literature review to determine the prevalence of peri-implant mucositis and peri-implantitis. For studies to be included in their assessment, patients needed to have been monitored more than 5 years and included more than 50 subjects. Only two investigations met these criteria. The data were reported with regard to the percentage of implants and percentage of patients who manifested peri-implant diseases. The investigators noted that after 5 years that peri-implant mucositis (bleeding upon probing) was found in approximately 80% of the subjects and around 50% of the implants. In the two groups included in the systematic review, peri-implantitis (bleeding and bone loss) was detected as follows: group 1-28% of the subjects and 12% of the sites: group 2-greater than 56% of subjects and at 43% of implant sites (Branemark implants [Nobel Biocare, CA, USA]). Accordingly, it can be concluded that over time the prevalence of peri-implant diseases is greater than previously expected.

Treatment for Peri-Implant Diseases

Nonsurgical therapy
Renvert and colleagues[68] selected 24 studies to assess nonsurgical therapy for mucositis and peri-implantitis. They reported that nonsurgical mechanical therapy could be used effectively to treat mucositis. Furthermore, antimicrobial mouth rinses improved the outcome of mechanical therapy. For peri-implantitis, however, nonsurgical therapy was not found to provide satisfactory outcomes, and adjunctive rinsing with chlorhexidine had limited value. Local or systemic drug delivery helped decrease

bleeding upon probing and probing depths[12,69–71]; however, it could not resolve peri-implantitis. They also indicated that laser therapy has the potential to be efficacious, but there are not enough data at this time to judge its effectiveness as a nonsurgical treatment modality.

Surgical therapy

Claffey and colleagues[72] evaluated information gathered from animal and human clinical trials concerning surgical therapy for peri-implantitis. Histologic data from animal studies validated that reosseointegration to contaminated surfaces was attainable, but not predictably.[72] No single method of decontaminating the roots (eg, chemical agents, air abrasives and lasers) appeared to be distinctly better than other techniques. It was concluded that open debridement with surface decontamination can resolve peri-implantitis (**Fig. 2**). With respect to people, one study indicated that therapy was successful in 58% of the patients.[73] Nevertheless, at present there does not appear to be a best treatment of peri-implantitis. Furthermore, bone grafts with and without barriers have been used with varying degrees of success.

A consensus statement from the 6th European Workshop on Periodontology found that for mucositis, nonsurgical mechanical therapy resulted in a reduction in

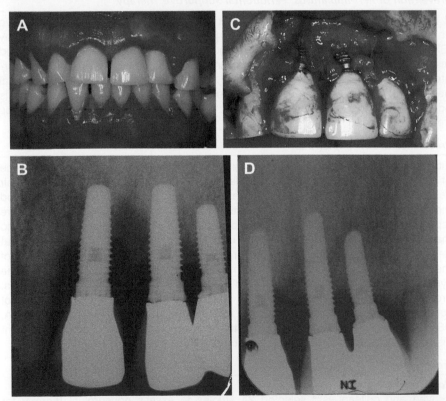

Fig. 2. (*A*) The patient presented with peri-implantitis at sites #s 9 through 11. (*B*) Radiograph of site #s 9 through 11 revealed bone loss around the dental implants. (*C*) Surgical debridement of infected dental implants. Debridement was coupled with decontamination of the implant surfaces with tetracycline. Then a bone graft and a barrier were placed. (*D*) One year postoperatively, the radiograph reveals some bone has been regenerated around the dental implants.

inflammation (bleeding on probing around implants) and that the adjunctive use of antimicrobial mouth rinses had a positive effect.[74] It was decided, however, that non-surgical treatment of peri-implantitis was unpredictable. The committee stated that the main reason for performing surgical treatment among patients with peri-implantitis was to attain access to the implant surface for debridement and decontamination to reduce the inflammatory lesion.

PROGNOSTICATION OF PERIODONTALLY COMPROMISED TEETH: A REQUIREMENT FOR TREATMENT PLANNING IMPLANT DENTISTRY

In this era of greater dental implant use, there is a propensity to misjudge the long-term prognosis of a tooth with a compromised periodontium (treated or untreated).[75–77] Thus, the practitioner may remove a tooth prematurely, reasoning that its retention can damage a potential implant site, or its inclusion in a prosthesis is too risky. Most studies, however, indicate that periodontally treated but questionable teeth have a better long-term retention rate (5 to 40 years) than expected (**Table 1**).[78–84]

Several recent review papers have noted that there is no single clinical parameter (eg, probing depth, bone loss, clinical attachment loss, mobility, or furcation invasion) that can dependably predict periodontal disease activity, tooth loss, or conversely, long-term tooth preservation.[75,77] Therefore, combinations of parameters need to be evaluated in concert with clinical judgment to plan treatment and to predict therapeutic outcomes. Furthermore, there is no accurate way to denote a threshold for tooth removal based on periodontal status that is correct in every circumstance. Accordingly, the judgment to remove a tooth will vary depending on its clinical status, and this endeavor should be supported by the best available literature, clinical experience, and the patient's declared goals. **Table 2** lists factors to consider when contemplating extraction versus retention of questionable teeth.[75]

Table 1
Term retention of questionable teeth: retrospective studies

Retrospective Studies	Number of Patients	Mean Years (Range) in Maintenance Treatment	Number of Teeth Assigned a Questionable Prognosis	Number of Questionable Teeth Retained During Maintenance	Number of Questionable Teeth Extracted During Maintenance
Becker et al[78]	95	5	120	89 (74%)	31 (26%)
Hirschfeld and Wasserman[79]	600	22 (15–53)	2,139	1473 (69%)	666 (31%)
McFall[80]	100	19 (15–29)	215	81 (38%)	134 (62%)
Mcleod et al[81]	114	12.5 (5–29)	907	781 (86%)	126 (14%)
Chace and Low[82]	166	40	455	400 (88%)	55 (12%)
Checchi et al[83]	92	6.7 (3–12)	578	557 (96%)	21 (4%)
Fardal et al[84]	100	9.8 (9–11)	346	335 (97%)	11 (3%)

Reprinted from Greenstein G, Greenstein B, Cavallaro J. Prerequisite for treatment planning implant dentistry: periodontal prognostication of compromised teeth. Compend Comp Cont Dent Ed 2007;28(8):436–47; with permission.

Table 2
Factors to consider when contemplating extraction versus retention of questionable teeth

Factor	Retention	Extraction of Teeth
Patient's wishes		
Caries		
Caries susceptibility	Not prone	Prone
Caries present	Minor	Extensive
Restorability	Easy	Difficult
Monetary issues	Retain	
Crown lengthening		
Esthetic zone	Low smile line	High smile line
Randomized control trial (RCT) needed		Probably removal
Periodontal status		
Periodontal attitude	Accepts surgery option	Does not want surgery
Maintenance compliance	Good	Poor
Bone levels		
Bone graft will help save tooth	Retain	
Additional bone loss ruins implant site		Remove
Bone level <10 mm	Caution needed	
Mobility		
Stability	Easy to stabilize	Requires extensive stabilization
Patient comfort	Patient comfortable	Patient uncomfortable
Root-resected teeth		Remove
Systemic issues (eg, valve replacement)		Remove
Furcations	Class 1 or 2 or 3	Class III (if poor oral hygiene)
Endodontic status		
Straight-forward RCT	Retain	
Re-treatment		Remove
Apicoectomy needed		Remove
Apical pathosis		Probably remove
Intact arch		
No prosthetic plan	Retain	
Complex prosthetic plan		Remove
Prosthetics		
Partial needed	Stabilizes questionable teeth	Rests on questionable teeth
Other implants	Provide occlusal stability	
Esthetic zone	Esthetics not a concern	If additional bone loss will make it unesthetic
Patient's attitude	Opposed to implants	
Seeking final solution		Remove questionable teeth
Dental history		
Abscesses	None or once	Multiple times
Surgical therapy	None or once	Multiple times

From Greenstein G, Greenstein B, Cavallaro J. Prerequisite for treatment planning implant dentistry: periodontal prognostication of compromised teeth. Compend Comp Cont Dent Ed 2007;28(8):436–47; with permission.

PERIODONTAL AND RESTORATIVE CONSIDERATIONS IN THE ESTHETIC ZONE IN PERIODONTAL PATIENTS

Numerous factors need to be considered when deciding whether to save or extract a tooth in the esthetic zone. These include restorability, disease susceptibility (caries and periodontitis), papillary and gingival considerations, tooth esthetics, smile line, the need for endodontic therapy, and the emotional and esthetic concerns of the patient. The decision to extract or maintain teeth must include deliberation with regard to benefits versus risks of retaining compromised teeth. The judgment to remove a tooth may be based on one critical issue or it may rely on collective risks related to a few factors.

SIZE OF PERIODONTAL DEFECTS

Typically, it is advantageous to preserve shallow rather than deep probing depths around teeth or implants.[85] A common outcome of periodontal surgery is gingival and papillary recession, however, this may result in unattractive black triangles between teeth. Thus, resective therapy that produces an unattractive gingival contour is contraindicated on teeth with a guarded prognosis in the esthetic zone.[86] In the premaxilla, it is sensible to remove periodontally questionable teeth and replace them with implants if this will aid in preserving the level of the gingiva and bone. Nevertheless, a result of preserving the gingival height where bone loss occurred is the need to accept deeper probing depths around implants when they are inserted, or the obligation to rebuild bone support before implants are placed (site development).

SUMMARY

The periodontal patient who has been treated and is receiving periodontal supportive therapy can be a candidate to receive dental implants if there are no systemic contraindications for therapy. In these individuals, implants can be placed in native bone, grafted bone, or in a sinus that has been augmented with bone. There should not be a rush to judgment with respect to removing periodontally compromised teeth and replacing them with dental implants, because these teeth often have better long-term prognoses than perceived by the dentist. On the other hand, in the esthetic zone, consideration should be given to removing teeth before altering the gingival topography and creating an esthetic dilemma. Ultimately, in the periodontal patient, it is a judgment call by the clinician that determines which teeth to retain and which to replace with dental implants. This decision needs to be based upon available scientific evidence, clinical experience of the clinician, dental history of the patient, and his or her desires.

REFERENCES

1. American Academy of Periodontology–Research, Science, and Therapy Committee; American Academy of Pediatric Dentistry. Treatment of plaque-induced gingivitis, chronic periodontitis, and other clinical conditions. Pediatr Dent 2005–2006;27(Suppl 7):202–11.
2. Ong CT, Ivanovski S, Needleman IG, et al. Systematic review of implant outcomes in treated periodontitis subjects. J Clin Periodontol 2008;35(5):438–62.
3. Mericske-Stern R. Prosthetic considerations. Aust Dent J 2008;53(Suppl 1): S49–59.
4. Caldas AF Jr. Reasons for tooth extraction in a Brazilian population. Int Dent J 2000;50(5):267–73.

5. Bailit HL, Braun R, Maryniuk GA, et al. Is periodontal disease the primary cause of tooth extraction in adults? J Am Dent Assoc 1987;114(1):40–5.
6. Murray H, Locker D, Kay EJ. Patterns of and reasons for tooth extractions in general dental practice in Ontario, Canada. Community Dent Oral Epidemiol 1996;24(3):196–200.
7. Reich E, Hiller KA. Reasons for tooth extraction in the western states of Germany. Community Dent Oral Epidemiol 1993;21(6):379–83.
8. Phipps KR, Stevens VJ. Relative contribution of caries and periodontal disease in adult tooth loss for an HMO dental population. J Public Health Dent 1995;55(4): 250–2.
9. Al-Shammari KF, Al-Khabbaz AK, Al-Ansari JM, et al. Risk indicators for tooth loss due to periodontal disease. J Periodontol 2005;76(11):1910–8.
10. Becker W, Becker BE, Berg LE. Periodontal treatment without maintenance. A retrospective study in 44 patients. J Periodontol 1984;55(9):505–9.
11. Tonetti MS, Steffen P, Muller-Campanile V, et al. Initial extractions and tooth loss during supportive care in a periodontal population seeking comprehensive care. J Clin Periodontol 2000;27(11):824–31.
12. Mombelli A. Microbiology and antimicrobial therapy of peri-implantitis. Periodontol 2000 2002;28:177–89.
13. Paster BJ, Boches SK, Galvin JL, et al. Bacterial diversity in human subgingival plaque. J Bacteriol 2001;183(12):3770–83.
14. Dharmar S, Yoshida K, Adachi Y, et al. Subgingival microbial flora associated with Brånemark implants. Int J Oral Maxillofac Implants 1994;9(3):314–8.
15. Silverstein LH, Kurtzman D, Garnick JJ, et al. The microbiota of the peri-implant region in health and disease. Implant Dent 1994;3(3):170–4.
16. Eke PI, Braswell LD, Fritz ME. Microbiota associated with experimental peri-implantitis and periodontitis in adult Macaca mulatta monkeys. J Periodontol 1998;69(2):190–4.
17. Mombelli A, Feloutzis A, Bragger U, et al. Treatment of peri-implantitis by local delivery of tetracycline. Clinical, microbiological and radiological results. Clin Oral Implants Res 2001;12(4):287–94.
18. Quirynen M, De Soete M, van Steenberghe D. Infectious risks for oral implants: a review of the literature. Clin Oral Implants Res 2002;13(1):1–19.
19. Shibli JA, Melo L, Ferrari DS, et al. Composition of supra- and subgingival biofilm of subjects with healthy and diseased implants. Clin Oral Implants Res 2008; 19(10):975–82.
20. Quirynen M, Vogels R, Peeters W, et al. Dynamics of initial subgingival colonization of pristine peri-implant pockets. Clin Oral Implants Res 2006;17(1):25–37.
21. Danser MM, van Winkelhoff AJ, van der Velden U. Periodontal bacteria colonizing oral mucous membranes in edentulous patients wearing dental implants. J Periodontol 1997;68(3):209–16.
22. Emrani J, Chee W, Slots J. Bacterial colonization of oral implants from nondental sources. Clin Implant Dent Relat Res 2009;11(2):106–12.
23. Devides SL, Franco AT. Evaluation of peri-implant microbiota using the polymerase chain reaction in completely edentulous patients before and after placement of implant-supported prostheses submitted to immediate load. Int J Oral Maxillofac Implants 2006;21(2):262–9.
24. Greenstein G, Lamster I. Bacterial transmission in periodontal diseases: a critical review. J Periodontol 1997;68(5):421–31.
25. Gafan GP, Lucas VS, Roberts GJ, et al. Prevalence of periodontal pathogens in dental plaque of children. J Clin Microbiol 2004;42(9):4141–6.

26. Karoussis IK, Kotsovilis S, Fourmousis I. A comprehensive and critical review of dental implant prognosis in periodontally compromised partially edentulous patients. Clin Oral Implants Res 2007;18(6):669–79.
27. Astrand P, Ahlqvist J, Gunne J, et al. Implant treatment of patients with edentulous jaws: a 20-year follow-up. Clin Implant Dent Relat Res 2008;10(4):207–17.
28. Adell R, Eriksson B, Lekholm U, et al. A long-term follow-up study of osseointegrated implants in the treatment of totally edentulous jaws. Int J Oral Maxillofac Implants 1990;5(4):347–59.
29. Jemt T, Johansson J. Implant treatment in the edentulous maxillae: a 15-year follow-up study on 76 consecutive patients provided with fixed prostheses. Clin Implant Dent Relat Res 2006;8(2):61–9.
30. Al-Zahrani MS. Implant therapy in aggressive periodontitis patients: a systematic review and clinical implications. Quintessence Int 2008;39:211–5.
31. Hämmerle CH, Jung RE, Feloutzis A. A systematic review of the survival of implants in bone sites augmented with barrier membranes (guided bone regeneration) in partially edentulous patients. J Clin Periodontol 2002;29(Suppl 3): 226–33.
32. Ellegaard B, Olsen-Petersen J, Baelum V. Implant therapy involving maxillary sinus lift in periodontally compromised patients. Clin Oral Implants Res 1997; 8(4):305–15.
33. Ellegaard B, Baelum V, Olsen-Petersen J. Nongrafted sinus implants in periodontally compromised patients: a time-to-event analysis. Clin Oral Implants Res 2006;17(2):156–64.
34. Zitzmann NU, Berglundh T. Definition and prevalence of peri-implant diseases. J Clin Periodontol 2008;35(Suppl 8):286–91.
35. Atassi F. Peri-implant probing: positives and negatives. Implant Dent 2002;11(4): 356–62.
36. Schou S, Holmstrup P, Reibel J, et al. Ligature-induced marginal inflammation around osseointegrated implants and ankylosed teeth: stereologic and histologic observations in cynomolgus monkeys (*Macaca fascicularis*). J Periodontol 1993; 64(6):529–37.
37. Etter TH, Håkanson I, Lang NP, et al. Healing after standardized clinical probing of the perlimplant soft tissue seal: a histomorphometric study in dogs. Clin Oral Implants Res 2002;13(6):571–80.
38. Heitz-Mayfield LJ. Peri-implant diseases: diagnosis and risk indicators. J Clin Periodontol 2008;35(Suppl 8):292–304.
39. Lang NP, Wetzel AC, Stich H, et al. Histologic probe penetration in healthy and inflamed peri-implant tissues. Clin Oral Implants Res 1994;5(4):191–201.
40. Jepsen S, Rühling A, Jepsen K, et al. Progressive peri-implantitis. Incidence and prediction of peri-implant attachment loss. Clin Oral Implants Res 1996;7(2): 133–42.
41. Sonick M, Abrahams J, Faiella RA. A comparison of the accuracy of periapical, panoramic, and computerized tomographic radiographs in locating the mandibular canal. Int J Oral Maxillofac Implants 1994;9(4):455–60.
42. De Smet E, Jacobs R, Gijbels F, et al. The accuracy and reliability of radiographic methods for the assessment of marginal bone level around oral implants. Dentomaxillofac Radiol 2002;31(3):176–81.
43. Azari A, Nikzad S. Computer-assisted implantology: historical background and potential outcomes-a review. Int J Med Robot 2008;4(2):95–104.
44. Tischler M. In-office cone beam computerized tomography: technology review and clinical examples. Dent Today 2008;27(6):102–6.

45. Roos-Jansåker AM, Renvert H, Lindahl C, et al. Nine- to fourteen-year follow-up of implant treatment. Part III: factors associated with peri-implant lesions. J Clin Periodontol 2006;33(4):296–301.
46. Ferreira SD, Silva GL, Cortelli JR, et al. Prevalence and risk variables for peri-implant disease in Brazilian subjects. J Clin Periodontol 2006;33(12):929–35.
47. Huynh-Ba G, Lang NP, Tonetti MS, et al. Association of the composite IL-1 geno-type with peri-implantitis: a systematic review. Clin Oral Implants Res 2008; 19(11):1154–62.
48. Strietzel FP, Reichart PA, Kale A, et al. Smoking interferes with the prognosis of dental implant treatment: a systematic review and meta-analysis. J Clin Periodon-tol 2007;34(6):523–44.
49. Lindquist LW, Carlsson GE, Jemt T. Association between marginal bone loss around osseointegrated mandibular implants and smoking habits: a 10-year follow-up study. J Dent Res 1997;76(10):1667–74.
50. Yeung SC. Biological basis for soft tissue management in implant dentistry. Aust Dent J 2008;53(Suppl 1):S39–42.
51. Block MS, Gardiner D, Kent JN, et al. Hydroxyapatite-coated cylindrical implants in the posterior mandible: 10-year observations. Int J Oral Maxillofac Implants 1996;11(5):626–33.
52. Bouri A Jr, Bissada N, Al-Zahrani MS, et al. Width of keratinized gingiva and the health status of the supporting tissues around dental implants. Int J Oral Maxillo-fac Implants 2008;23(2):323–6.
53. Kim BS, Kim YK, Yun PY, et al. Evaluation of peri-implant tissue response accord-ing to the presence of keratinized mucosa. Oral Surg Oral Med Oral Pathol Oral Radiol Endod 2009;107(3):e24–8.
54. Wennström JL, Bengazi F, Lekholm U. The influence of the masticatory mucosa on the peri-implant soft tissue condition. Clin Oral Implants Res 1994;5(1):1–8.
55. Zigdon H, Machtei EE. The dimensions of keratinized mucosa around implants affect clinical and immunological parameters. Clin Oral Implants Res 2008; 19(4):387–92.
56. Cairo F, Pagliaro U, Nieri M. Soft tissue management at implant sites. J Clin Periodontol 2008;35(Suppl 8):163–7.
57. Bengazi F, Wennström JL, Lekholm U. Recession of the soft tissue margin at oral implants. A 2-year longitudinal prospective study. Clin Oral Implants Res 1996; 7(4):303–10.
58. Chung DM, Oh TJ, Shotwell JL, et al. Significance of keratinized mucosa in main-tenance of dental implants with different surfaces. J Periodontol 2006;77(8): 1410–20.
59. Albrektsson T, Zarb G, Worthington P, et al. The long-term efficacy of currently used dental implants: a review and proposed criteria of success. Int J Oral Max-illofac Implants 1986;1(1):11–25.
60. Teughels W, Van Assche N, Sliepen I, et al. Effect of material characteristics and/ or surface topography on biofilms development. Clin Oral Implants Res 2006; 17(Suppl 2):68–81.
61. Berglundh T, Gotfredsen K, Zitzmann NU, et al. Spontaneous progression of liga-ture induced peri-implantitis at implants with different surface roughness: an experimental study in dogs. Clin Oral Implants Res 2007;18(5):655–61.
62. Martines RT, Sendyk WR, Gromatzky A, et al. Sandblasted/acid-etched vs smooth-surface implants: implant clinical reaction to xperimentally induced peri-implantitis in Beagle dogs. J Oral Implantol 2008;34(4):185–9.

63. Astrand P, Engquist B, Anzén B, et al. A three-year follow-up report of a comparative study of ITI dental implants and Brånemark system implants in the treatment of the partially edentulous maxilla. Clin Implant Dent Relat Res 2004;6(3): 130–41.

64. Wennström JL, Ekestubbe A, Gröndahl K, et al. Oral rehabilitation with implant-supported fixed partial dentures in periodontitis-susceptible subjects. A 5-year prospective study. J Clin Periodontol 2004;31(9):713–24.

65. Albouy JP, Abrahamsson I, Persson LG, et al. Spontaneous progression of peri-implantitis at different types of implants. An experimental study in dogs. I: clinical and radiographic observations. Clin Oral Implants Res 2008;19(10):997–1002.

66. Quirynen M, Abarca M, Van Assche N, et al. Impact of supportive periodontal therapy and implant surface roughness on implant outcome in patients with a history of periodontitis. J Clin Periodontol 2007;34(9):805–15.

67. Cohen RE, Research, Science and Therapy Committee, American Academy of Periodontology. Position paper: periodontal maintenance. J Periodontol 2003; 74(9):1395–401.

68. Renvert S, Roos-Jansåker AM, Claffey N. Non-surgical treatment of peri-implant mucositis and peri-implantitis: a literature review. J Clin Periodontol 2008; 35(Suppl 8):305–15.

69. Renvert S, Lessem J, Dahlén G, et al. Mechanical and repeated antimicrobial therapy using a local drug delivery system in the treatment of peri-implantitis: a randomized clinical trial. J Periodontol 2008;79(5):836–44.

70. Salvi GE, Persson GR, Heitz-Mayfield LJ, et al. Adjunctive local antibiotic therapy in the treatment of peri-implantitis II: clinical and radiographic outcomes. Clin Oral Implants Res 2007;18(3):281–5.

71. Büchter A, Meyer U, Kruse-Lösler B, et al. Sustained release of doxycycline for the treatment of peri-implantitis: randomised controlled trial. Br J Oral Maxillofac Surg 2004;42(5):439–44.

72. Claffey N, Clarke E, Polyzois I, et al. Surgical treatment of peri-implantitis. J Clin Periodontol 2008;35(Suppl 8):316–32.

73. Leonhardt A, Dahlén G, Renvert S. Five-year clinical, microbiological, and radiological outcome following treatment of peri-implantitis in man. J Periodontol 2003; 74(10):1415–22.

74. Lindhe J, Meyle J, Group D of European Workshop on Periodontology. Peri-implant Diseases: consensus report of the sixth European workshop on periodontology. J Clin Periodontol 2008;35(Suppl 8):282–5.

75. Greenstein G, Greenstein B, Cavallaro J. Prerequisite for treatment planning implant dentistry: periodontal prognostication of compromised teeth. Compend Contin Educ Dent 2007;28(8):436–47.

76. McGuire MK, Nunn ME. Prognosis versus actual outcome. II. The effectiveness of clinical parameters in developing an accurate prognosis. J Periodontol 1996; 67(7):658–65.

77. Avila G, Galindo-Moreno P, Soehren S, et al. A novel decision-making process for tooth retention or extraction. J Periodontol 2009;80(3):476–91.

78. Becker W, Berg L, Becker B. The long-term evaluation of periodontal treatment and maintenance in 95 patients. Int J Periodontics Restorative Dent 1984;4(2): 54–71.

79. Hirschfeld L, Wasserman B. A long-term survey of tooth loss in 600 treated periodontal patients. J Periodontol 1978;49(5):225–37.

80. McFall W. Tooth loss in 100 treated patients with periodontal disease. A long-term study. J Periodontol 1982;53(9):539–49.

81. McLeod D, Phillip L, Spivey J. The effectiveness or periodontal treatment as measured by tooth loss. J Am Dent Assoc 1997;128(3):316–24.
82. Chace R Sr, Low SB. Survival characteristics of periodontally involved teeth: a 40 year study. J Periodontol 1993;64(8):701–5.
83. Checchi L, Montevecchi M, Gatto MR, et al. Retrospective study of tooth loss in 92 treated periodontal patients. J Clin Periodontol 2002;29(7):651–6.
84. Fardal O, Johannessen AC, Linden G. Tooth loss during maintenance following periodontal treatment in a periodontal practice in Norway. J Clin Periodontol 2004;31(7):550–5.
85. Greenstein G. Diagnostic and therapeutic implications of increased probing depths: current interpretations. Compend Contin Educ Dent 2005;26(6):381–90.
86. Greenstein G, Cavallaro J, Tarnow D. When to save or extract a tooth in the esthetic zone: a commentary. Compend Contin Educ Dent 2008;29(6):136–47.

Treatment of Gingival Recession

Moawia M. Kassab, DDS, MS[a],*, Hala Badawi, DDS[b],
Andrew R. Dentino, DDS, PhD[a]

KEYWORDS

- Gingival recession • Gingival grafting
- Connective tissue grafting • Guided tissue regeneration
- Coronally positioned flap

Gingival recession is an intriguing and complex phenomenon. Recession frequently disturbs patients because of sensitivity and esthetics. Many surgical techniques have been introduced to treat gingival recession, including those involving autogenous tissue grafting, various flap designs, orthodontics, and guided tissue regeneration (GTR). This article describes different clinical approaches to treat gingival recession with emphasis on techniques that show promising results and root coverage.

ETIOLOGY AND PREVALENCE

Recession can be defined as the displacement of the gingival margin apically from the cementoenamel junction (CEJ), or from the former location of the CEJ where restorations have distorted the location or appearance of the CEJ. Gingival recession can be localized or generalized, and be associated with one or more surfaces.[1]

Many people exhibit generalized gingival recession without any awareness of the condition and without symptoms. However, patients are often anxious about gingival recession for one or several reasons, including fear of tooth loss, dentinal hypersensitivity, or poor esthetics. Because many possible contributing factors interact to contribute to gingival recession, it is difficult to predict whether further changes in gingival recession may occur at a given site.

Albandar and Kingman[2] studied the prevalence of gingival recession among subjects 30 to 90 years old. Using a sample of 9689 subjects, they projected that 23.8 million persons in the United States have one or more tooth surfaces with 3 mm or more gingival recession. Those investigators also found that the prevalence of 1 mm or more recession in persons 30 years and older was 58%, and increased with age. Males had significantly more gingival recession than females, and African

[a] Department of Surgical Sciences, Marquette University, School of Dentistry, PO Box 1881, Milwaukee, WI 53201-1881, USA
[b] Marquette University, School of Dentistry, PO Box 1881, Milwaukee, WI 53201-1881, USA
* Corresponding author.
E-mail address: moe.kassab@marquette.edu (M.M. Kassab).

Dent Clin N Am 54 (2010) 129–140
doi:10.1016/j.cden.2009.08.009
0011-8532/09/$ – see front matter Crown Copyright © 2010 Published by Elsevier Inc. All rights reserved.

Americans had significantly more gingival recession than members of other racial/ethnic groups. Recession also was more prevalent and severe at buccal than at interproximal surfaces of teeth.[2] Similarly, Gorman[3] found that the frequency of gingival recession increased with age, and was greater in males than females of the same age. Malpositioned teeth and toothbrush trauma were found to be the most frequent etiologic factors associated with gingival recession.[3] Recession associated with labially positioned teeth occurred in 40% of patients 16 to 25 years old, and increased to 80% of patients in the 36- to 86-year-old group.[3] Those findings were corroborated by Gorman,[4] who examined 4000 subjects and found that the incidence of gingival recession increased with age.

The indications for surgical treatment of gingival recession include reducing root sensitivity, minimizing cervical root caries, increasing the zone of attached gingiva, and improving esthetics.

CONNECTIVE TISSUE GRAFTING

One goal of soft tissue grafting is root coverage. To accomplish that goal, many techniques and flap designs have been used, some of which do not require a donor site (pedicle grafts), while others do (free autogenous grafts). The success rates of root coverage procedures vary because coverage depends on several factors, including location and classification of the gingival recession and the technique used. The gingival dimension most commonly assessed is the height (distance between the soft tissue margin and the mucogingival line measured in millimeters). An increase in gingival height independent of the number of millimeters is considered a successful outcome of gingival augmentation procedures.[5]

PEDICLE GRAFTS

Pedicle grafts differ from free autogenous soft tissue grafts in that the base of the pedicle flap contains its own blood supply, which nourishes the graft and facilitates the reestablishment of vascular union with the recipient site. Pedicle grafts may be partial or full thickness.[6,7] In a clinical human study, Wood and colleagues[8] used reentry procedures to compare crestal radicular bone responses to full- and partial-thickness flaps. He concluded that regardless of the flap procedure, loss of crestal bone depended on thickness, with the thinnest radicular bone associated with greater postoperative bone loss. The mean bone loss for full- and partial-thickness flaps was 0.62 mm and 0.98 mm, respectively.

The term *lateral sliding flap* was first introduced by Grupe and Warren.[9] Miller and Allen[10] have noted that that term now generally refers to the laterally positioned pedicle graft (LPPG). An LPPG cannot be performed unless there is significant gingiva lateral to the site of recession. A shallow vestibule also may jeopardize outcomes. Although the use of the LPPG provides an ideal color match, it often is inadequate for the treatment of multiple recessions.

Pedicle grafts using an edentulous area as a donor site also have been proposed to correct gingival recession.[11] The procedure is particularly useful in cases where the attached gingiva on facial surfaces of two or three consecutive teeth is inadequate. That technique involves the development of partial-thickness flaps around the involved teeth, sliding the entire flap the width of half a tooth, and placing the interdental papillary tissues over the buccal surfaces of the affected teeth.[12]

Cohen and Ross[13] proposed a double-papilla repositioned flap to cover defects where an insufficient amount of gingiva was present, or where there was an inadequate amount of gingiva in an adjacent area for a lateral sliding flap. The papillae from each side of the tooth are reflected and rotated over the midfacial aspect of the recipient tooth and sutured. The only advantage of this technique is the dual blood supply and denudation only of interdental bone. The disadvantages may include pulling of the sutures and tearing of the gingival papilla.[13–15]

Coronally Positioned Grafts

Bernimoulin and colleagues[16] first described the coronally positioned graft subsequent to grafting with a free graft (ie, a two-stage procedure).

First, a free autogenous soft tissue graft is placed apical to an area of denuded root. After healing, the flap is coronally repositioned. The requirements for the success of coronally positioned grafts include (1) the presence of shallow crevicular depths on proximal surfaces, (2) approximately normal interproximal bone heights, (3) tissue height within 1 mm of the CEJ on adjacent teeth, (4) adequate healing of the free graft before coronal positioning, (5) reduction of any root prominence within the plane of the adjacent alveolar bone, and (6) adequate release of the flap to prevent retraction during healing. The second-stage procedure uses a split-thickness dissection with mesial and distal vertical releasing incisions until adequate flap mobility is obtained. The flap is sutured 0.5 to 1 mm coronal to the CEJ and covered with a periodontal dressing.[17]

Coronally positioned flaps were compared with lateral sliding flaps in the treatment of localized gingival recessions.[18,19] In a 6-month report, both techniques rendered satisfactory results, and no differences in tissue coverage, sulcus depth, or gain of attached gingiva were reported. An average of 2.7 mm of soft tissue coverage was obtained, with average recession coverage of 67%. The only difference between the two techniques was an increase in root exposure of approximately 1 mm at the lateral sliding flap donor site, while no additional recession was observed with the coronally positioned flap. Results were stable for 3 years.

Allen and Miller[20] used single-stage coronally positioned flaps in the treatment of shallow marginal recession. The Miller class I defects had a minimum keratinized tissue width of 3 mm, with recession between 2.5 to 4 mm. The technique consisted of citric acid root treatment, a split-thickness flap extending into the vestibule, and surface gingivoplasty of the papillae to produce a bleeding bed. Flaps were sutured into position and dressed. Complete root coverage was attained in 84% of the sites, with a mean root coverage gain of 3.2 mm. Similarly, Harris[21] reported a 98% success rate of root coverage in class I defects by using the coronally positioned graft technique.

Tarnow[22] described the semilunar coronally positioned flap technique. An incision is made that follows the curvature of the free marginal gingiva and extends into the papillae, staying at least 2 mm from the papilla tip on either side. The incision is made far enough apically to ensure that the apical portion of the flap rests on bone after repositioning. A split-thickness dissection of the flap is made and the flap is repositioned and held in place with light pressure and a periodontal dressing. The advantages of that technique include no tension on the flap after repositioning, no shortening of the vestibule, no reflection of the papillae (thereby avoiding esthetic compromise), and no suturing.

FREE AUTOGENOUS SOFT TISSUE GRAFTS

Both the epithelialized palatal graft and the subepithelial connective tissue graft offer a more versatile solution for root coverage than does the laterally positioned or coronally positioned pedicle flaps. There is adequate donor tissue, a shallow vestibule does not compromise the procedure, and multiple recessions can be treated. Two kinds of autogenous grafts can be used for root coverage. One consists of an epithelialized layer, while the other does not (or contains a small epithelialized collar).

Free Epithelialized Autogenous Gingival Grafts

Sullivan and Atkins[23] were the first to explore the feasibility and healing of the free gingival graft. This procedure involves the preparation of a recipient site, which is accomplished by supraperiosteal dissection to remove epithelium and connective tissue to the periosteum.

Some of the common areas for donor material include edentulous ridges, attached gingiva, and palatal gingiva. Because of shrinkage during healing, donor tissue should be approximately 33% larger than the anticipated healed graft.[24] The grafts used should be approximately 0.8 to 1.3 mm in thickness to assure that there is an adequate connective tissue component.[25]

In a 2-year study comparing graft versus no graft, plaque control was more important than the width of the attached gingiva in determining eventual breakdown and recession.[26] Investigators also found that the use of the free gingival graft was a predictable means of increasing the width of the attached gingiva. In a follow-up study 2 years later, the same investigators reported similar results except that 10% of the nongrafted cases showed additional soft tissue recession compared with grafted sites with equivalent plaque scores.[27]

Free gingival grafting has been used as a single procedure to cover denuded root surfaces.[28] The recipient bed is extended one tooth-width lateral to the denuded roots, and 5 mm apical to the gingival margin of the denuded root. The investigators suggested that donor tissue cover the gingival bed and extend at least 3 mm apical to the margin of the denuded root, using a graft of approximately 1.5 mm uniform thickness. In 50 randomly selected cases, recessions less than 3 mm had 95.5% root coverage, recessions 3 to 5 mm had 80.6% coverage, and recessions more than 5 mm had 76.6% coverage.

Miller[29] described a technique for root coverage using a free soft tissue autograft with citric acid treatment. Predictable root coverage depended upon the severity and classification of gingival recession. After root planing, citric acid application was performed, followed by horizontal incisions at the level of the CEJ to preserve the interdental papillae. Vertical incisions at proximal line angles of adjacent teeth facilitate completion of bed preparation. A thick palatal graft with a thin layer of submucosa was placed on a moderately bleeding bed and stabilized with sutures at the papillary and apical ends of the graft extending into periosteum. Results of 100 consecutively placed grafts showed 100% root coverage in class I defects and 88% coverage in class II. The average root coverage for all sites was 3.8 mm with a mean clinical attachment gain of 4.5 mm.

Although Miller reported a combined 90% success rate in achieving 100% root coverage, his 100 cases included 94 in the mandible and only 6 in the maxilla.

Connective Tissue Autogenous Grafts

The use of connective tissue grafts for root coverage was first reported by Langer and Langer.[30] A partial-thickness flap with two vertical incisions was elevated on the recipient site, followed by placement of the graft (which is collected from the palate by a double parallel incision technique). The flap is coronally positioned to attempt to cover the graft and benefit from a double blood supply. They reported an increase of 2 to 6 mm of root coverage in 56 cases over 4 years.

Raetzke[31] described an envelope technique for obtaining root coverage using connective tissue grafts. In that technique, the collar of marginal tissue around a localized area of recession is excised, the root is debrided and planed, and a split-thickness envelope created around the denuded root surface. The graft was collected from the palate by means of the double parallel incision technique. The connective tissue graft is placed in the previously created envelope covering the exposed root surface. Overall, 80% of the exposed root surfaces were covered. Similarly, Allen[32] reported an 84% success rate for root coverage using that same technique.

Jahnke and colleagues[33] compared the results of free gingival and connective tissue grafts for root coverage in nine patients. Paired defects were selected and assessed preoperatively, as well as 3 and 6 months postoperatively. Root coverage averaged for 43% for the free gingival graft group, and 80% for the connective tissue graft group. Borghetti and Louise,[34] in their split-mouth controlled clinical study, reported a 70% success rate of root coverage 1 year postoperatively.

Most of the studies that used the connective tissue grafts for root coverage did not attempt to remove the epithelial collar from the graft, but when Bouchard and colleagues[35] did so, no additional statistically significant benefits were observed (65% with collar, 70% without).

When the connective tissue graft was compared with the free gingival graft for root coverage, Paolantonio and colleagues[36] found in a 5-year postoperative study that the connective tissue graft provided a predictable percentage of root coverage (85%), while the free gingival graft presented only a 53% success rate. They concluded that connective tissue grafting is a long-term predictable procedure for root coverage.

A variety of techniques have been used to collect the connective tissue graft, including parallel incisions and free gingival knife methods with no significant difference in the percentage of root coverage.[37]

COMBINATION OF ONE OR MORE TECHNIQUES

To increase the success rate of root coverage, many clinicians have attempted to combine different procedures (**Figs. 1–5**). Nelson[38] used connective tissue grafting with a double pedicle graft. A free connective tissue graft first was placed over the

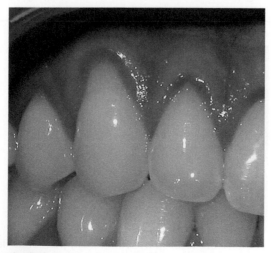

Fig. 1. Preoperative gingival recession on tooth #6.

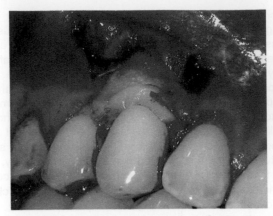

Fig. 2. Connective tissue graft sutured in place around tooth #6.

denuded root surface, followed by a double pedicle graft to partially cover the connective tissue graft. Twenty-nine defects were treated with that technique and monitored for 4 years. The mean root coverage was 88% (7–10 mm of recession), 92% (4–6 mm of recession), and 100% (≤3 mm of recession). Harris[14] modified Nelson's technique with a split-thickness pedicle graft to cover the connective tissue graft. Thirty Miller class I and II defects were selected and the mean root coverage was 97%.

Wennström and Zucchelli[5] compared a coronally positioned flap to a combination of a coronally positioned and connective tissue graft procedure. The treatment of 103 (Miller class I and II) defects was performed. The success rate for the combination group was 98.9%, while 97% was accomplished for the control group after a 2-year postoperative evaluation. The investigators concluded that the previous combination of coronally positioned flap and connective tissue graft was the treatment of choice to achieve root coverage.

Recent studies report that the addition of platelet-rich plasma to the combination of connective tissue grafting and coronally positioned grafts revealed no additional clinical benefits.[39,40] Allografts have also been tested to treat gingival recession and to

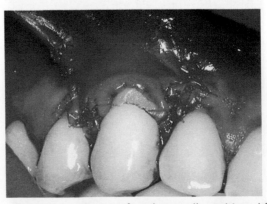

Fig. 3. Combination of connective tissue graft and coronally positioned flap with sutures at tooth #6.

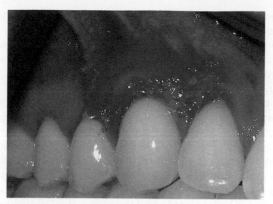

Fig. 4. Tooth #6 after 2 weeks of postoperative healing.

eliminate the donor site. Results appear to be contradictory, possibly because the procedure is technique sensitive, especially when aimed at root coverage.[41,42]

Various tissue engineering techniques, including those involving the use of enamel matrix derivative, have been used to enhance root coverage. However, minimal clinical significance has been reported in terms of root coverage.[43-45]

GUIDED TISSUE REGENERATION (GTR) TO TREAT GINGIVAL RECESSION

Regeneration is defined as "a reproduction or reconstitution of a lost or injured part. It is, therefore, the biologic process by which the architecture and function of lost tissues are completely restored."[15] This implies regeneration of the tooth's supporting tissues, including alveolar bone, periodontal ligament, and cementum. Many studies have attempted to achieve regeneration, but success rates have varied from minimal or partial regeneration to almost complete regeneration.

The use of GTR has been suggested for treatment of recession. Tinti and Vincenzi[46] first reported a case where GTR using an expanded polytetrafluoroethylene (ePTFE) membrane was used to treat recession defects. Cortellini, Clauser, and Pini Prato[47] also demonstrated, histologically, that the root coverage obtained with an ePTFE membrane included new connective tissue attachment as well as new bone formation.

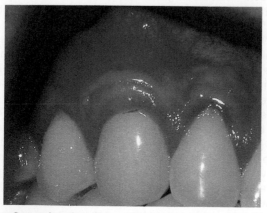

Fig. 5. Tooth #6 after 6 months of postoperative healing.

Different space-making solutions also have been used in combination with nonresorbable membranes (eg, titanium-reinforced, gold bar–reinforced, and gold frame–reinforced membranes) to increase the percentage of root coverage with GTR. In a human histologic study using titanium-reinforced membranes, there was evidence of new connective tissue attachment and new bone growth after 9 months.[48] The different membrane designs have resulted in 77% root coverage.[49]

Roccuzzo and colleagues[50] used ePTFE membranes in combination with miniscrews for space-making and stabilization, reporting a mean root coverage of 84% in 12 cases. Jepsen and colleagues[51] compared titanium-reinforced membranes and connective tissue grafts using the envelope technique. There was no statistically significant difference in the two treatment modalities (the mean root coverage was 87% for the GTR group and 86% for the connective tissue graft group). Wang and colleagues[52] also compared GTR to subepithelial connective tissue grafting. Using 16 patients with bilateral Miller class I and II recession, they concluded that both treatments presented with statistically significant improvement from preoperative to postoperative measurements. The mean root coverage for the GTR group was 73%, and 84% for the subepithelial connective tissue graft.

To eliminate the need for a second surgical procedure to remove a nonresorbable membrane, the use of various bioabsorbable materials has been proposed. In one study, root coverage was obtained using a bioabsorbable polylactic acid membrane softened with citric acid ester (PLACA membrane).[53] In another study, the PLACA membrane resulted in a mean root coverage of 64%.[54] In comparing the use of a PLACA membrane to a nonresorbable ePTFE membrane, investigators found no statistically significant differences in the mean root coverage obtained by either technique (PLACA 82%; ePTFE 83%).[50] Similarly, Zucchelli and colleagues[55] showed similar results when they compared bioabsorbable to nonabsorbable membranes.

The choice of GTR or gingival grafting to obtain root coverage has been a controversial subject. For example, Pini Prato and colleagues[56] compared the results obtained with ePTFE membrane and a two-step mucogingival surgical procedure (involving a free gingival graft and coronally positioned flap). They reported mean root coverage for the GTR procedure of 72% versus mean root coverage for the two-step procedure of 70% (the differences were not statistically significant). Harris[57] also compared GTR with a bioabsorbable membrane versus connective tissue with double pedicle graft, and the difference was not statistically significant.

The combination of coronally positioned flap procedures and GTR was assessed in a clinical investigation.[58] The investigators found in their 6-month split-mouth randomized design that there was no statistically significant difference between GTR/coronally positioned flaps versus coronally positioned flaps alone. The mean root coverage was 56% and 69%, respectively. Another study reported similar results, with no statistically significant differences observed between the two treatment groups.[59] However, the later study reported a slight increase in the width of keratinized gingiva in the connective tissue group. Ricci and colleagues[60] also showed similar results after a 1-year postoperative evaluation, with no statistically significant differences between treatments (77% mean root coverage for the GTR group and 80% for the connective tissue group). Harris[61] combined a connective tissue graft with a coronally positioned graft and compared it to GTR with a bioabsorbable membrane. No differences were observed between groups (92% for the GTR group and 95% for the connective tissue with coronally positioned graft). He also noticed a greater increase in the amount of keratinized gingival tissue for the connective tissue graft group. Trombelli and colleagues[62] showed a significant difference in mean root coverage when comparing the GTR with a bioabsorbable membrane to a connective tissue graft procedure (48% root coverage for the GTR group and 81% root coverage for the connective tissue graft), and reported a significant increase in the amount of keratinized gingival tissue for the connective tissue graft when compared with the GTR group. However, in a more recent study,[63] when GTR was compared with connective tissue grafting with coronally positioned flaps, the investigators concluded that, in shallow recessions (1.5 to 3.5 mm), GTR techniques only provided 50% root coverage obtained 12 months postoperatively, while the connective tissue grafting techniques yielded 82% root coverage. Harris[64] supported the previous conclusion by reporting that 92% mean root coverage obtained 6 months postoperatively had been reduced to a 58% after a mean of 25 months' postoperative evaluation.

SUMMARY

The treatment of gingival recession can be accomplished with a variety of procedures. However, the combination of connective tissue grafting with a coronally positioned flap has been shown to demonstrate the highest success rate. Allograft materials and GTR techniques also can be used to treat recessions, particularly when patients are reluctant to consent to providing gingiva donor sites.

REFERENCES

1. Smith RG. Gingival recession. Reappraisal of an enigmatic condition and a new index for monitoring. J Clin Periodontol 1997;24:201–5.
2. Albandar JM, Kingman A. Gingival recession, gingival bleeding, and dental calculus in adults 30 years of age and older in the United States, 1988–1944. J Periodontol 1999;70:30–43.
3. Gorman WJ. The prevalence and etiology of gingival recession. J Periodontol 1967;38:316–22.
4. Murray JJ. Gingival recession in tooth types in high fluoride and low fluoride areas. J Periodont Res 1973;8:243–53.
5. Wennström JL, Zucchelli J. Increased gingival dimensions. A significant factor for successful outcome of root coverage procedures. A 2 year prospective clinical study. J Clin Periodontol 1996;23:770–7.
6. Pfeifer J, Heller R. Histologic evaluation of full and partial thickness lateral repositioned flaps: a pilot study. J Periodontol 1971;42:331–3.
7. Sugarman EF. A clinical and histologic study of the attachment of grafted tissue to bone and teeth. J Periodontol 1969;40:381–7.
8. Wood DL, Hoag FM, Donnenfeld OW, et al. Alveolar crest reduction following full and partial thickness flaps. J Periodontol 1972;43:141–4.
9. Grupe HE, Warren RF. Repair of gingival defects by a sliding flap operation. J Periodontol 1956;27:290–5.
10. Miller PD, Allen EP. The development of periodontal plastic surgery. Periodontol 2000 1996;11:7–17.
11. Corn H. Edentulous area pedicle grafts in mucogingival surgery. J Periodontol 1964;2:229–42.
12. Hattler AB. Mucogingival surgery utilization of interdental gingival as attached gingiva by surgical displacement. J Periodontol 1967;5:126–31.
13. Cohen DW, Ross SE. The double papillae repositioned flap in periodontics. J Periodontol 1968;39:65–70.
14. Harris RJ. The connective tissue and partial thickness double pedicle graft: a predictable method of obtaining root coverage. J Periodontol 1992;63: 477–86.

15. The American Academy of Periodontology. Annals of periodontology world workshop in periodontics. vol. 1. num. 1. Chicago (IL): The American Academy of Periodontology, Journal of Periodontology; 1996. p. 621.
16. Bernimoulin JP, Luscher B, Muhlemann H. Coronally repositioned periodontal flap. J Clin Periodontol 1975;2:1–13.
17. Maynard JG. Coronal positioning of a previously placed autogenous gingival graft. J Periodontol 1977;48:151–5.
18. Guinard EA, Caffesse RG. Treatment of local recession. Part III. Comparison of results obtained with lateral sliding and coronally repositioned graft. J Periodontol 1978;49:457–61.
19. Caffesse RG, Guinard EA. Treatment of localized recessions. Part IV. Results after three years. J Periodontol 1980;51:167–70.
20. Allen EP, Miller PD. Coronal positioning of existing gingiva: short-term results in the treatment of shallow marginal tissue recession. J Periodontol 1989;60:316–9.
21. Harris RJ. The connective tissue with partial thickness double pedicle graft. The result of 100 consecutively treated defects. J Periodontol 1994;65:448–61.
22. Tarnow DP. Semilunar coronally repositioned flap. J Clin Periodontol 1986;13: 182–5.
23. Sullivan HC, Atkins JH. Free autogenous gingival grafts. III. Utilization of grafts in the treatment of gingival recession. J Periodontol 1968;6:152–9.
24. Egli U, Vollmer W, Rateikschaick KH. Followup studies of free gingival grafts. J Clin Periodontol 1975;2:98–104.
25. Soehren SE, Alien AL, Cutright DE, et al. Clinical and histologic studies of donor tissue utilized for free grafts of masticatory mucosa. J Periodontol 1973;44:727–41.
26. Dorfman HS, Kennedy JE, Bird WC. Longitudinal evaluation of free gingival autografts. J Clin Periodontol 1980;7:316–24.
27. Dorfman HS, Kennedy JE, Bird WC. Longitudinal study of free autogenous gingival grafts. A 4-year report. J Periodontol 1982;53:349–52.
28. Holbrook T, Ochsenbein C. Complete coverage of the denuded root surface with a one stage gingival graft. Int J Periodontics Restorative Dent 1983; 3(3):9–27.
29. Miller PD. Root coverage using the free soft tissue autograft following citric acid application. III. A successful and predictable procedure in areas of deep wide recession. Int J Periodontics Restorative Dent 1985;5(2):15–37.
30. Langer B, Langer L. Subepithelial connective tissue graft technique for root coverage. J Periodontol 1985;56:715–20.
31. Raetzke P. Covering localized areas of root exposure employing the "envelope" technique. J Periodontol 1985;56:397–402.
32. Allen AL. Use of the supraperiosteal envelop in the soft tissue grafting for root coverage. II. Clinical results. Int J Periodontics Restorative Dent 1994;14:303–15.
33. Jahnke PV, Sandifer JP, Gher ME, et al. Thick free gingival graft and connective tissue autografts for root coverage. J Periodontol 1993;64:315–22.
34. Borghetti A, Louis F. Controlled clinical evaluation of the subpedicle connective tissue graft for the coverage of gingival recession. J Periodontol 1994;65: 1107–12.
35. Bouchard P, Etienne D, Ouhayoun J, et al. Subepithelial connective tissue grafts in the treatment of gingival recession. A comparative study of 2 procedures. J Periodontol 1994;65:929–36.
36. Paolantonio M, Muro C, Cattabriga A, et al. Subpedicle connective tissue graft versus free gingival graft in the coverage of exposed root surfaces. A 5 year clinical study. J Clin Periodontol 1997;24:51–6.

37. Harris RJ. A comparison of two techniques for obtaining a connective tissue graft from the palate. Int J Periodontics Restorative Dent 1997;17:261–71.
38. Nelson S. The subpedicle connective tissue graft. A bilaminar reconstructive procedure for the coverage of denuded root surfaces. J Periodontol 1986;95:102.
39. Petrungaro PS. Using platelet-rich plasma to accelerate soft tissue maturation in esthetic periodontal surgery. Compend Contin Educ Dent 2001;22:729–32.
40. Huang LH, Neiva RE, Soehren SE, et al. The effect of platelet-rich plasma on the coronally advanced flap root coverage procedure: a pilot human trial. J Periodontol 2005;76:1768–77.
41. Harris RJ. A comparative study of root coverage obtained with an acellular dermal matrix versus a connective tissue graft: results of 107 recession defects in 50 consecutively treated patients. Int J Periodontics Restorative Dent 2000; 20:51–9.
42. Papageorgakopoulos G, Greenwell H, Hill M, et al. Root coverage using acellular dermal matrix and comparing a coronally positioned tunnel to a coronally positioned flap approach. J Periodontol 2008;79(6):1022–30.
43. McGuire MK, Nunn M. Evaluation of human recession defects treated with coronally advanced flaps and either enamel matrix derivative or connective tissue. Part 1: comparison of clinical parameters. J Periodontol 2003;74:1110–25.
44. McGuire MK, Nunn ME. Evaluation of the safety and efficacy of periodontal applications of a living tissue-engineered human fibroblast-derived dermal substitute. I. Comparison to the gingival autograft: a randomized controlled pilot study. J Periodontol 2005;76:867–80.
45. McGuire MK, Scheyer ET, Nunn ME, et al. A pilot study to evaluate a tissue-engineered bilayered cell therapy as an alternative to tissue from the palate. J Periodontol 2008;3:1847–56.
46. Tinti C, Vincenzi G. The treatment of gingival recession with guided tissue regeneration procedure by means of Gore-Tex membranes. Quintessence Int 1990;6: 465–8.
47. Cortellini P, Clauser C, Pini Prato G. Histological assessment of new attachment following the treatment of a human buccal recession by means of a guided tissue regeneration procedure. J Periodontol 1993;64:387–91.
48. Parma-Benfenati S, Tinti C. Histologic evaluation of new attachment utilizing a titanium-reinforced barrier membrane in a mucogingival recession defect. A case report. J Periodontol 1998;69:834–9.
49. Tinti C, Vincenzi G, Cocchetto R. Guided tissue regeneration in mucogingival surgery. J Periodontol 1993;64:1184–91.
50. Roccuzzo M, Lungo M, Corrente G, et al. Comparative study of a bioresorbable and a non-resorbable membrane in the treatment of human recessions. J Periodontol 1996;67:7–14.
51. Jepsen K, Heimz B, Halben H, et al. Treatment of gingival recession with titanium reinforced barrier membranes versus connective tissue grafts. J Periodontol 1998;69:383–91.
52. Wang HL, Bunyaratavej P, Labadie M, et al. Comparison of 2 clinical techniques for treatment of gingival recession. J Periodontol 2001;72(10):1301–11.
53. Genon P, Genon-Romagna C, Gottlow J. Treatment of gingival recessions with guided tissue regeneration: a bioresorbable barrier. J Periodontol Implantol Orale 1994;13:289–96.
54. Pini Prato G, Clauser C, Magnani C, et al. Resorbable membranes in the treatment of human buccal recession: a nine-case report. Int J Periodontics Restorative Dent 1995;15:258–67.

55. Zucchelli G, Clauser C, De Sanctis M, et al. Mucogingival versus guided tissue regeneration procedures in the treatment of deep recession type defects. J Periodontol 1998;69:138–45.
56. Pini Prato G, Tinti C, Vincenzi G, et al. Guided tissue regeneration versus mucogingival surgery in the treatment of human buccal recession. J Periodontol 1992; 63:919–28.
57. Harris RJ. A comparative study of root coverage obtained with guided tissue regeneration utilizing a bioabsorbable membrane versus the connective tissue with partial-thickness double pedicle graft. J Periodontol 1997;68:779–90.
58. Amarante ES, Leknes KN, Skavland J, et al. Coronally positioned flap procedure with or without a bioabsorbable membrane in the treatment of human gingival recession. J Periodontol 2000;71:989–98.
59. Borghetti A, Glise J, Monnet-Corti V, et al. Comparative clinical study of a bioabsorbable membrane and subepithelial connective tissue graft in the treatment of human gingival recession. J Periodontol 1999;70:123–30.
60. Ricci G, Silvestri M, Tinti C, et al. A clinical/statistical comparison between the subpedicle connective tissue graft method and the guided tissue regeneration technique in root coverage. Int J Periodontics Restorative Dent 1996;16:538–45.
61. Harris RJ. A comparison of 2 root coverage techniques: guided tissue regeneration with a bioabsorbable matrix style membrane versus a connective tissue graft combined with a coronally positioned pedicle graft without vertical incisions. Results of series of consecutive cases. J Periodontol 1998;69:1426–34.
62. Trombelli L, Scabbia A, Tatakis DN, et al. Subpedicle connective tissue graft versus guided tissue regeneration with bioabsorbable membrane in the treatment of human gingival recession defects. J Periodontol 1998;69:1271–7.
63. Muller HP, Stahl M, Eger T. Failure of root coverage of shallow gingival recessions employing GTR and bioresorbable membrane. Int J Periodontics Restorative Dent 2001;21:171–81.
64. Harris RJ. GTR for root coverage: a long-term follow-up. Int J Periodontics Restorative Dent 2002;22:55–61.

Future Approaches in Periodontal Regeneration: Gene Therapy, Stem Cells, and RNA Interference

Giuseppe Intini, DDS, PhD

KEYWORDS

- Periodontal therapy • Periodontal regeneration
- Gene therapy • RNA interference • Stem cells

Periodontal disease is characterized by inflammation that leads to alveolar bone loss and destruction of periodontal ligament. Epidemiologic research shows that approximately 50% of the adult population between the ages of 45 and 65 years have periodontal disease.[1] Recent scientific evidence highlights the connection between periodontitis and the pathogenesis or maintenance of other diseases.[2–6] Periodontal disease is a public health issue and the development of effective therapies to treat periodontal disease and regenerate periodontal tissue is a major goal of the scientific community.

The challenges in regenerative periodontal therapy lie in the ability to induce the regeneration of a complex apparatus composed of different tissues, such as bone, cementum, and periodontal ligament. Despite the recent advancements in periodontal therapy,[7,8] a complete regeneration of the damaged periodontium is still unattainable. Various therapeutic approaches, including the use of recombinant growth factors, have been applied and none of them have been shown to induce complete regeneration of the lost periodontium.

The regeneration of the periodontal tissue is no different in principle from the regeneration of any other body tissue. Currently, there are five main types of therapeutics used or in development for tissue regeneration: (1) conductive therapeutics, (2) inductive therapeutics, (3) cell-based therapeutics, (4) gene-based therapeutics, and (5) RNA-based therapeutics.[9–12]

A conductive therapeutic is a biocompatible scaffold that guides the regeneration of the tissue by passively allowing the attachment and growth of vascular elements and

Department of Developmental Biology, Harvard School of Dental Medicine, 188 Longwood Avenue, REB 513, Boston, MA 02115, USA
E-mail address: giuseppe_intini@hsdm.harvard.edu

Dent Clin N Am 54 (2010) 141–155
doi:10.1016/j.cden.2009.09.002
0011-8532/09/$ – see front matter © 2010 Elsevier Inc. All rights reserved.

progenitor stem cells that reside in the tissue defect. Its regenerative potential is limited by the lack of biologically active factors and sufficient progenitor cells within the defect. Examples of conductive therapeutics for periodontal regeneration are hydroxyapatite, tricalcium phosphate, and calcium sulfate fillers.

An inductive therapeutic is a biocompatible scaffold that guides and induces the regeneration of the tissue by carrying one or more biologically active factors that recruit vascular elements and progenitor stem cells from the immediate vicinity to the tissue defect. Its regenerative potential is higher than the conductive biomaterial because more progenitor cells can repopulate the tissue defect. Examples of inductive therapeutics for periodontal regeneration are allogenic bone grafts or biomaterials carrying osteoinductive recombinant proteins.

A cell-based therapeutic is a biocompatible scaffold that contains progenitor stem cells or differentiated cells. The cells are delivered within the tissue defect and become tissue-forming cells. Bone autografts may be considered as cell-based therapeutics for periodontal regeneration. As the result of stem cell research, cell-based therapeutics has been proposed for the delivery of undifferentiated or partially differentiated progenitor cells. Theoretically, the regenerative potential of a stem cell–based therapy is the highest, but limited by the scarce availability of sources for cells.

A gene-based therapeutic is a biocompatible scaffold carrying single or multiple genes that transform the nonprogenitor cells already present within the tissue defect into both progenitor and mature tissue-specific cells. As such, a gene therapy product does not need to carry and deliver progenitor cells within the tissue defect. Rather, it is able to signal the cells present in the defect to differentiate into a phenotype more favorable to the regeneration process, and it represents an attractive solution for regenerative therapy.

Because of their enormous potential, RNA-based therapeutics may be considered a fifth category of regeneration therapy even though this approach remains in a conceptual stage of development. They are based on the principle of RNA interference (RNAi), a novel mechanism of action by which RNAs silence gene expression. Novel therapeutic approaches may be envisioned whereby the expression of certain genes detrimental to the tissue regeneration process is silenced by RNAs.

This article analyzes the advances made by the scientific community in terms of periodontal regeneration, mainly focusing on gene-based and stem cell–based therapeutics. Additionally, the potential for RNAi as a new tool in modern regenerative biology is discussed.

GENE THERAPY
The Biology of Gene Therapy

The gene therapy approach to tissue regeneration presents the advantage of potentially mimicking the complex natural process of tissue formation. One or more genes encoding for growth factors or transcriptional regulators may be delivered within the tissue defect, fostering the regeneration of the missing tissue. These factors may be delivered simultaneously or sequentially to control the timing and distribution of the delivered factors,[10,13,14] resembling their expression during the healing process.

Most studies of gene therapy for tissue regeneration have been conducted using either adenovirus vectors, adenoassociated viruses, retroviruses, lentiviruses, or naked DNA.[10,15] Adenoviruses have the advantage of not depending on cell replication for the delivery of DNA. In addition, adenoviral DNA does not normally integrate into the host genome. For this reason, the transgene expression from adenoviruses is quite brief (up to 2 weeks according to some recent research).[16] Cells infected by adenoviruses may secrete viral proteins, however, and elicit an undesired immune response. In contrast, adenoassociated viruses do not express viral proteins and are nonimmunogenic. They can infect dividing and nondividing cells without integrating into the genome and provide transient gene expression.[10] Yet, adenoassociated viruses are difficult to construct because their development requires helper viruses that make purification problematic.

Retroviruses are the most extensively used vectors for applications in gene therapy. They are RNA viruses that, thanks to the viral enzyme reverse transcriptase, make a DNA copy of their genome, which can randomly integrate into the host cell genome. Replication-incompetent murine leukemia virus, which is nonpathogenic in humans, is the most used among retroviruses for gene therapy. Murine leukemia virus exists in host cells only as DNA and is unable to transcribe genes encoding viral coat proteins. Murine leukemia virus cannot elicit an immune response. As observed in recent clinical trials,[17,18] however, the integrated retrovirus can disrupt the host DNA by insertional mutagenesis, producing serious adverse effects. In addition, because the virus is permanently integrated into the genome, the induced gene expression also is permanent. This phenomenon is not ideal for such transitory processes as periodontal regeneration and tissue regeneration in general.

Lentiviruses are a specialized form of retroviruses that have the advantage of infecting nondividing cells. Also, host genome integration seems to be more limited and less random than retroviruses, limiting the possibility of insertional mutagenesis.[19] Lentiviruses are derived from pathogenic viruses, however, such as HIV-1, and may not be considered safe for clinical use. More importantly, they may provide a continuous expression of the transgene and may not be suitable for temporary regenerative processes.

For all the previously mentioned reasons, viral gene therapy may not be the most suitable gene therapy approach for tissue regeneration. Indeed, naked DNA for nonviral gene therapy is easier and cheaper to manufacture, is available on a large scale, is less immunogenic, presents a low likelihood of being inserted into the cell genome, and allows for transient expression of the transgene.[10,20,21] Unfortunately, the transfection efficiency of naked DNA is extremely low and naked DNA remains elusive and ineligible for tissue regeneration and gene therapy in general. For this reason, several researchers have tried to complex the naked DNA in different chemical formulations to increase cellular DNA uptake and subsequent gene expression. In particular, cationic and anionic liposomes have been shown to increase the uptake of DNA in tissue culture cells and in vivo.[22,23] Yet, as currently formulated, the transfection of cells by naked DNA is an inefficient process, with an estimated efficiency of 10^{-9} that of viral vectors.[24] Novel approaches have introduced the concept of passive uptake of naked DNA. By this method, the DNA molecules are immobilized in vivo by carriers, such as collagen[25,26] or polymer matrices,[27] to form the so-called "gene-activated matrices." The immobilized DNA is then up-taken by the cells. Because the DNA stays in place for a longer time, the transfection efficiency is increased. By this technique, between 30% and 50% of the cell population exposed to the DNA expresses the transgene and the transfection is higher when compared with previous in vivo approaches.[25–27]

Gene Therapy for Periodontal Regeneration

The efficacy of gene-based therapeutics for periodontal regeneration has been demonstrated only in preclinical studies, where viral approaches have been shown to have potential. Some of the most interesting studies in this field have been performed using viral vectors encoding for platelet-derived growth factor (PDGF).[28] Initial investigations found that adenoviral vectors effectively transduced osteoblasts, cementoblasts, periodontal ligament cells, and gingival fibroblasts to induce the expression of PDGF in vitro.[29,30] It was demonstrated that on viral transduction, the expression of PDGF was maintained for up to 10 days in human gingival fibroblasts.[31] Subsequently, the feasibility of in vivo delivery of PDGF by adenoviral gene transfer to stimulate periodontal tissue regeneration in large tooth-associated alveolar bone defects in rats was demonstrated.[32] An adenoviral vector encoding bone morphogenetic protein (BMP)-7 for regeneration of periodontal defects in rats was also successfully used,[33] indicating that other growth factors may be effective in periodontal regenerative gene therapy.

Others have investigated the ability of adenoviral vectors to induce bone formation in bone defects. For instance, Lieberman and colleagues[34] used an ex vivo approach to create BMP-2 producing bone marrow cells. The bone marrow cells producing BMP-2 were successfully used to heal a critical size femoral segmental defect in rats. Delivery of BMP-2 by adenoviral vector also proved to be successful in bone healing of segmental defects created in the femora of New Zealand rabbits[35] and in regeneration of other bone defects.[36–38] Recently, a combinatorial approach was successfully tested in cells transduced with adenoviruses encoding both BMP-2 and BMP-7.[39] These cells were more effective in healing cranial defects than were cells individually transduced with adenoviruses encoding either BMP-2 or BMP-7.

Retroviruses have also been investigated as potential and effective vectors for bone regeneration. For instance, the ability of a retroviral expression vector encoding for sonic hedgehog to induce regeneration of bone was demonstrated in rat calvaria critical size defects.[40] Retroviral vectors were also successfully used to transduce skeletal muscle cells, inducing them to express human BMP-2. These cells, once implanted into critical size calvaria defects in mice, induced a full closure of the defect by 8 weeks.[41]

One of the most promising gene therapy approaches for periodontal regeneration is based on the combination of naked DNA with a biodegradable carrier.[25–27] Using this approach, collagen or other carriers are used to engineer a so-called "gene-activated matrix" (GAM) that can carry and deliver the naked DNA in vivo. An elegant demonstration that this method can be used for bone regenerative therapy comes from the pioneering studies of Bonadio and coworkers.[26] In their work, a plasmid encoding for the N-terminal fragment of the human parathyroid hormone was physically entrapped in a collagen matrix sponge and implanted into a critical size canine skeletal defect. This gene-activated collagen matrix induced bone regeneration in a stable, reproducible, and dose-dependent manner.

The GAM approach was later used by others for alternative gene therapy studies. For instance, plasmids that encode basic fibroblast growth factor-2, brain-derived neurotrophic factor, and neurotrophin-3 entrapped in GAM were shown to promote sustained survival of retinal ganglion cells for over 3 months after a central nervous system injury in rats.[42] More recently, a study showed that angiogenesis and osteogenesis can be promoted by a GAM carrying a plasmid encoding for human vascular endothelial growth factor (VEGF) in atrophic bone nonunion defects in rabbits.[43] Others[44] have used a plasmid encoding transforming growth factors-ss1 entrapped in GAM fabricated with chitosan and gelatin to induce cartilage regeneration into cartilage defects of rabbit knee joints. In this study the authors achieved new cartilage formation and concluded that this therapeutic protocol provided a cost-effective, simple, and efficient method for repair of cartilage defects. Another recent work reports that modifying GAM with calcium-phosphate precipitates enhances the efficiency of the in vivo gene transfer.[45] This study showed that the modified GAM carrying a plasmid encoding human BMP-2 is more efficient than the traditional GAM in inducing bone regeneration in a critical size segmental bone defect in rat tibiae.

Clearly, the nonviral approach using GAM has the potential to offer transient but efficient delivery of a specific gene that is suitable for periodontal regenerative therapy. Unfortunately, despite the high transfection efficiency observable, GAM still requires an enormous amount of plasmid DNA to achieve some therapeutic effect. The previously mentioned studies use plasmid amounts in the range of 1 to 100 mg, depending on the size of the bone defects. Moreover, difficulties in the preparation of collagen-based GAMs may limit its clinical use.[10,20,21]

Gene therapy presents certain advantages when compared with other therapies. Because both cell transplantation and laboratory cell culturing are not needed, gene therapy may be safer and more cost-effective than cell-based therapies.[10] Moreover, when compared with the existing recombinant single-protein–based therapies,[7,46] gene therapy may mimic the complex natural process of periodontal tissue formation, because multiple genes, and multiple factors, can be delivered within the bone defect.[10,13,14]

Since the inception of gene therapy (mid- to late-1980s), researchers have launched more than 400 clinical trials, testing the approach against a wide spectrum of diseases. The Food and Drug Administration, however, has recently declared that "little has worked"[47] and more studies are needed to improve gene therapy. Despite some successes, several tragic outcomes, such as treatment-induced cancers and death caused by allergic reactions, have hampered and derailed the field.[47] The encouraging findings of the previously mentioned studies may promote more much needed basic research with the final goal of developing effective and safer gene-based therapeutics.

STEM CELLS
Stem Cell Biology

The most relevant limitation of biomaterials available for tissue regeneration is their lack of promotion or delivery of competent cells to the site where tissue repair is required, resulting in inadequate regeneration. To overcome this problem, researchers are focusing their efforts on the use of stem cells to be delivered within the tissue defect.

A stem cell is a clonogenic (able to form colonies in cultures), undifferentiated cell that is capable of differentiating into a different phenotype. Stem cells that differentiate into any cell type from all the three germ layers of the body (ectoderm, endoderm, and mesoderm) are defined as "pluripotent" stem cells. In contrast, stem cells that can differentiate into a cell type from only one or two germ layers are defined as "multipotent."[48] In general, three categories of stem cells can be identified: (1) embryonic stem cells (pluripotent); (2) adult stem cells (multipotent); and (3) reprogrammed stem cells (either pluripotent or multipotent).

Embryonic stem cells are derived from the inner cell mass of the blastocyst.[49] In culture they are able to form teratomas, agglomerations of cells with phenotypic characteristics of cell types from all the three germ layers of the body. There is still a plethora of concerns associated with their use in clinical therapies, including ethical concerns and biologic obstacles, such as their potential for tumorigenesis.[49,50]

Adult stem cells have been isolated from many specialized tissues, including bone marrow, epithelium, adipose tissue, liver, and the nervous system,[51–55] and may represent a safer approach to stem cell–based tissue regeneration. Because of their limited number and the technical difficulties related to their isolation and expansion, however, currently adult stem cells are used in few clinical applications. For instance, hematopoietic stem cells are used to treat lymphomas[56,57] and bone marrow stromal stem cells have been shown to be successful in regenerating bone in animal[58–60] and preclinical human studies.[61,62]

Reprogrammed stem cells are defined as cells whose genetic program has been substituted or modified to induce a switch from one cell phenotype to another phenotype.[63] Cell reprogramming is a challenging and yet fascinating goal for today's regenerative medicine because reprogrammed cells may serve as a valuable and safe tool for tissue engineering.

There are four routes by which cell reprogramming can be achieved. The first, defined as nuclear transfer from somatic cells to eggs and oocytes, is achieved by transferring a viable cell nucleus into an enucleated egg (**Fig. 1**). This method, first used for the creation of a cloned adult sheep (Dolly),[64] remains ethically controversial for human studies because it requires the explantation and the nuclear transplantation of an unfertilized oocyte.

The second and more viable route is represented by the pluripotency induced in somatic cells by the overexpression of certain genes or by modulation of certain signaling pathways (see **Fig. 1**). Takahashi and Yamanaka[65] at Kyoto University in Japan were the first to induce pluripotency in mouse fibroblasts by viral transduction of four genes named *Oct 3/4*, *Sox2*, *c-Myc*, and *KLF4*. These cells, named "induced pluripotent" stem (iPS) cells, show properties similar to those of embryonic stem cells.[66] Recent research has shown that *Oct 3/4* alone may be sufficient to induce

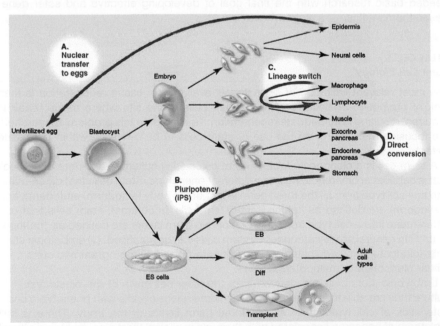

Fig. 1. Four possible routes to cell reprogramming. (A) Nuclear transfer from somatic cells to eggs and oocytes. (B) Pluripotency induced by overexpression of embryonic genes or by modulation of certain signaling pathways. (C) Lineage switching back to a branch point and out again in a different direction induced by tissue-specific genes. (D) Direct conversion induced by cell-specific genes. (*From* Gurdon JB, Melton DA. Nuclear reprogramming in cells. Science 2008;322:1811–5; with permission.)

pluripotency in somatic cells.[67] Opening the way to a safer approach to iPS cells, latest developments have shown the ability of nonviral methods, such as episomal vectors[68] or plasmid vectors,[69] to induce pluripotency in somatic cells. The modulation of certain signaling pathways induced by chemicals, such as valproic acid[70] or other small molecules,[71] is also being tested and may represent a safer alternative for the induction of iPS.

The third route to cell reprogramming is represented by lineage switching and is possible because of the discovery of so-called "master genes" (see **Fig. 1**).[63] For instance, the overexpression of the gene *MyoD* can induce a nonmuscle cell back to a partially undifferentiated state and then guide its maturation into a muscle cell.[72]

The fourth route is represented by direct conversion, a nonlineage switching of a cell into a different phenotype induced by specific genes (see **Fig. 1**). For instance, a recent study demonstrated the ability of three β-pancreas–specific genes to convert exocrine pancreas cells into insulin-producing pancreas β-cells.[73]

The improvement of the iPS technology, of lineage switching, and of direct conversion technologies could represent the most exciting line of research for the development of effective, safe, and ethically acceptable stem cell–based therapies.

Stem Cells for Periodontal Regeneration

Cell-based therapeutics for periodontal tissue regeneration may be engineered thanks to the latest developments in stem cell research. Although science is far from the use of iPS cells for the regeneration of periodontal tissue, for clinical practice, the use of adult stem cells and of reprogrammed stem cells by lineage switching or direct conversion may represent a promising and valid avenue for the future of periodontal therapeutics. To this end, researchers have recently focused their attention on the isolation and characterization of periodontal stem cells as common progenitors of fibroblasts, cementoblasts, and osteoblasts that form the tissues of the periodontium. For several years it has been known that cells derived from the periodontal ligament can differentiate into osteoblasts or cementoblasts to contribute to periodontal regeneration.[74–76] Direct evidence of the existence of a stem cell population within the periodontal tissue was found in 2004,[77] however, as multipotent periodontal ligament stem cells (PDLSC) were first isolated from the periodontal ligament of extracted teeth. These cells express mesenchymal stem cell markers, such as STRO-1 and MCAM (CD146), and were shown to be clonogenic and able to differentiate into adipocytes, osteoblasts, and cementoblast-like cells both in vitro and in vivo.[77–79] Using antibodies against STRO-1, MCAM, and CD44 Chen and colleagues[80] have identified and localized PDLSC in diseased and healthy periodontal human tissues. Recently PDLSC were also indentified in regenerating periodontal tissue, indicating that they directly contribute to periodontal regeneration.[81] PDLSC are very similar to other adult stem cells in that they are multipotent and clonogenic and express common markers, such as STRO-1 and MCAM. This similarity may also be detrimental, however, when it comes to isolation and expansion of PDLSC for the construction of cell-based therapeutics. This is because the use of antibodies against STRO-1 and MACM may result in the selection of a heterogeneous population of mesenchymal stem cells rather than a pure population of PDLSC. The challenge lies in the ability of identifying a PDLSC-specific marker that allows for the selection of a pure PDLSC population. Toward this end, researchers have been testing if these cells express markers, such as scleraxis, a tendon-specific transcription factor that may be expressed in higher concentrations in PDLSC because of their ability to form a ligament. Although PDLSC do express scleraxis in higher concentration when compared with bone-marrow derived and dental-pulp derived stem cells,[77] it is clear that this is not a unique marker for PDLSC.

Other efforts are under way to find an appropriate delivery system for engineering an efficient cell-based therapeutic tool for periodontal tissue regeneration.[82] Flores and colleagues[83] have found that fibrin gels carrying several layers of PDL cells (the so-called "cell sheet technique") can be successfully used as a delivery system for these cells, whereas Nakahara and colleagues[84] have successfully tested collagen sponge scaffolds seeded with PDL cells for the regeneration of periodontal fenestration defects in beagle dogs. Additionally, a delivery system for PDLSC based on a combination of bovine bone with human dentin was shown to be effective because these stem cells formed a cementum-like complex in subcutaneous dorsum pockets of immunocompromized mice.[85] Recently, platelet-rich plasma was also proposed as a putative carrier for adult stem cells into periodontal defects[86] and into larger bone defects.[87]

Enormous steps forward have been taken in the research of periodontal stem cells and cell delivery systems, leading to the promise of cell-based therapeutics for periodontal regeneration in the near future.

RNA INTERFERENCE
The Biology of RNAi

Thanks to the work of Andrew Fire and Craig Mellow, the mechanisms by which RNAs can silence gene expression are now understood[88] (for introductory information, see videos at http://www.arkitek.com/RNA_interference.html or at http://www.nature.com/focus/rnai/animations/index.html). The RNA-mediated silencing process is defined as RNAi, a discovery for which Fire and Mellow received the 2006 Nobel Prize. The discovery of RNAi has opened the door to RNA-based therapeutics that may prove to be an effective tool for the treatment of a large variety of diseases and for tissue regeneration, including periodontal tissue regeneration.[89]

RNAi works through small RNAs of approximately 20 to 30 nucleotides[90] that guide the degradation of complementary or semicomplementary molecules of messenger RNAs (posttranscriptional gene silencing) or interfere with the expression of certain genes at the promoter level (transcriptional gene silencing) (**Fig. 2**). Today, researchers can artificially induce RNAi by introducing synthetic molecules of RNA into cells.[89]

Artificially transcribed short hairpin RNAs (shRNAs) can be introduced into the cell by plasmid transfection or viral transduction, or small linear RNAs (siRNA) can be directly transfected into the cells.[91] In the cytoplasm, the shRNAs or siRNAs participate in endogenous posttranscriptional gene silencing. The synthetic RNAs are recognized and processed by an endoribonuclease named Dicer and incorporated into the RNA-induced silencing complex. Then, silencing occurs through the AGO2-mediated cleavage of target messenger RNAs (see **Fig. 2**).

Most RNA-based therapeutics currently under investigation use siRNAs because they are safer and more cost-effective than shRNAs. They can be introduced into the cells without the aid of viruses and can be chemically synthesized. The first siRNA-based therapeutic tested in human clinical trials was the VEGF-targeted RNA for the treatment of macular degeneration of the retina.[89] VEGF-targeted RNA is currently in phase III trials for the treatment of macular degeneration of the retina and in phase II for the treatment of diabetic macular edema. The directed ocular injection of siRNA against the VEGF receptor 1 was also recently tested and found to be effective in the reduction of neovascularization in mouse models of retinal and choroidal neovascularization.[92] This siRNA therapy is now in phase II clinical trials.

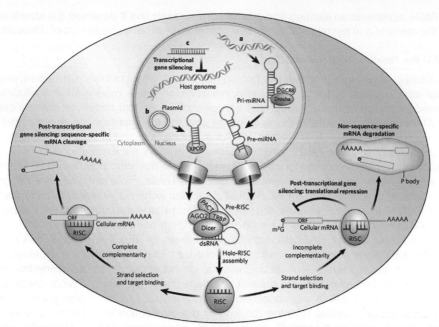

Fig. 2. (a) Mechanisms of the endogenous posttranscriptional RNA-mediated gene silencing. Primary microRNAs (pri-miRNAs) are processed by Drosha and DGCR8 into precursors miRNAs (pre-miRNAs). Pre-miRNAs are then transported into the cytoplasm by exportin 5 (XPO5). Once in the cytoplasm, they are bound and processed by a Dicer-containing pre–RNA-induced silencing complex (RISC) to form the so-called "holo-RISC," which contains all the components required to gene silencing, including AGO2, the catalytic core of the RISC complex. The miRNA that has been processed and is now bound to RISC, representing a guiding miRNA molecule of approximately 20–30 nucleotides that recognizes and binds the corresponding target RNA. At this point two things may happen: if the guiding miRNA is fully complementary to the target mRNA (*left pathway in the figure*), it triggers the catalysis of the target mRNA through AGO2; if the guiding miRNA is only partially complementary to the target mRNA (*right pathway in the figure*), a nonsequence specific degradation occurs in the P bodies. (b) Mechanisms of the artificially induced posttranscriptional gene silencing. Artificially transcribed shRNA may be introduced into the cell by plasmid transfection or viral transduction. These shRNA are then transported into the cytoplasm where they are recognized and processed by Dicer to form the RISC complex. Then, the silencing mechanism of action occurs through the AGO2-mediated cleavage. A similar mechanism of action is followed by small RNAs that may be directly transfected into the cells (siRNA). (c) Transcriptional RNA-mediated gene silencing. A not fully elucidate transcriptional silencing has been recently described and occurs when silencing RNAs are present into the nucleus and are complementary to the promoter regions of the genes. (*From* Castanotto D, Rossi JJ. The promises and pitfalls of RNA-interference-based therapeutics. Nature 2009;457:426–33; with permission.)

Another approach under investigation is a siRNA that targets an enzyme required for the synthesis of DNA as a possible strategy for the treatment of solid tumors.[89] The race for treatment of cancer with RNA-based therapeutics has just started.[93] For instance, Li and colleagues[94] have recently shown that a mixture of siRNA targeting MDM2, c-Myc, and VEGF transcripts injected into the bloodstream reduced by 70% to 80% the melanoma lung metastases in a mouse model.

RNAi represents an exciting and promising approach and it deserves the attention of the medical and dental community as a potential new tool for treatment of diseases.

RNAi for Periodontal Regeneration

As RNAi emerges as a promising technology for the treatment of several diseases, one may also envision RNAi to be an effective tool for tissue regeneration, including periodontal regeneration. Through the silencing of genes that negatively control cell proliferation and cell differentiation or genes that induce inflammation or apoptosis, RNAi may favor tissue regeneration.[11,12] For instance, a recent in vitro study showed that silencing the gene PHD2, which negatively regulates the expression of HIF1α in endothelial cells, favors the formation of microvessel-like structures and production of angiogenic factors by human umbilical endothelial cells.[11] The same siRNA strategy was later applied in vivo in a mouse model of cardiac ischemia, whereby mice treated with PHD2-targeted siRNA exhibited reduced infarct size when compared with saline-treated controls.[95] This strategy may be used to favor periodontal regeneration.

In an in vivo rat model of osteoarthritis, the delivery of NF-κB-targeted siRNA alleviates the inflammation of synovium and reduces the degradation of cartilage.[96] Cathepsin B–targeted siRNA also prevents chondrocytes from dedifferentiation, providing a potential tool to prevent cartilage degeneration.[97] Tumor necrosis factor-α–targeted siRNA can suppress osteolysis induced by metal particles in a murine calvaria model, opening the way to the application of RNAi in orthopedic and dental implant therapy.[98] In terms of bone regeneration, Gazzerro and colleagues[99] have demonstrated that down-regulation of Gremlin by RNAi in ST-2 stromal and MC3T3 osteoblastic cells increases the BMP-2 stimulatory effect on alkaline phosphatase activity and on Smad 1/5/8 phosphorylation, enhances osteocalcin and Runx-2 expression, and increases Wnt signaling, with the potential to increase bone formation in vivo. Taken together, these studies prove that RNAi, when adequately used, can foster tissue regeneration.

The use of RNA-based therapeutics for tissue regeneration is still in its early stages. Nevertheless, RNAi promises to be an effective therapeutic tool and may be successful in periodontal regeneration.

SUMMARY

This article highlights the recent scientific advancements in gene therapy, stem cell biology, and RNAi providing a summary of the ongoing research in these fields and identifying their potential in periodontal tissue regeneration. Results from basic research, preclinical, and clinical studies suggest that these fields of research may soon contribute to more effective therapies for periodontal regeneration.

ACKNOWLEDGMENT

The author is indebted to Joelle Carlo, PhD (Harvard School of Dental Medicine, Boston, MA), for the in-depth review of this manuscript.

REFERENCES

1. Oliver RC, Brown LJ, Loe H. Periodontal diseases in the United States population. J Periodontol 1998;69(2):269–78.
2. Scannapieco FA, Panesar M. Periodontitis and chronic kidney disease. J Periodontol 2008;79(9):1617–9.

3. Friedewald VE, Kornman KS, Beck JD, et al. The American Journal of Cardiology and Journal of Periodontology editors' consensus: periodontitis and atherosclerotic cardiovascular disease (diamond). J Periodontol 2009;80(7):1021–32.

4. Paju S, Scannapieco FA. Oral biofilms, periodontitis, and pulmonary infections. Oral Dis 2007;13(6):508–12.

5. Scannapieco FA. Systemic effects of periodontal diseases. Dent Clin North Am 2005;49(3):533–50, vi.

6. Tezal M, Sullivan MA, Reid ME, et al. Chronic periodontitis and the risk of tongue cancer. Arch Otolaryngol Head Neck Surg 2007;133(5):450–4.

7. Nevins M, Giannobile WV, McGuire MK, et al. Platelet-derived growth factor stimulates bone fill and rate of attachment level gain: results of a large multicenter randomized controlled trial. J Periodontol 2005;76(12):2205–15.

8. Taba M Jr, Jin Q, Sugai JV, et al. Current concepts in periodontal bioengineering. Orthod Craniofac Res 2005;8(4):292–302.

9. Salgado AJ, Coutinho OP, Reis RL. Bone tissue engineering: state of the art and future trends. Macromol Biosci 2004;4(8):743–65.

10. Franceschi RT. Biological approaches to bone regeneration by gene therapy. J Dent Res 2005;84(12):1093–103.

11. Cheema SK, Chen E, Shea LD, et al. Regulation and guidance of cell behavior for tissue regeneration via the siRNA mechanism. Wound Repair Regen 2007;15(3): 286–95.

12. Yao Y, Wang C, Varshney RR, et al. Antisense makes sense in engineered regenerative medicine. Pharm Res 2009;26(2):263–75.

13. Lattanzi W, Pola E, Pecorini G, et al. Gene therapy for in vivo bone formation: recent advances. Eur Rev Med Pharmacol Sci 2005;9(3):167–74.

14. Luo J, Sun MH, Kang Q, et al. Gene therapy for bone regeneration. Curr Gene Ther 2005;5(2):167–79.

15. Phillips JE, Gersbach CA, Garcia AJ. Virus-based gene therapy strategies for bone regeneration. Biomaterials 2007;28(2):211–29.

16. Zhao M, Zhao Z, Koh JT, et al. Combinatorial gene therapy for bone regeneration: cooperative interactions between adenovirus vectors expressing bone morphogenetic proteins 2, 4, and 7. J Cell Biochem 2005;95(1):1–16.

17. Hacein-Bey-Abina S, von Kalle C, Schmidt M, et al. A serious adverse event after successful gene therapy for X-linked severe combined immunodeficiency. N Engl J Med 2003;348(3):255–6.

18. Noguchi P. Risks and benefits of gene therapy. N Engl J Med 2003;348(3): 193–4.

19. Vigna E, Naldini L. Lentiviral vectors: excellent tools for experimental gene transfer and promising candidates for gene therapy. J Gene Med 2000;2(5): 308–16.

20. Partridge KA, Oreffo RO. Gene delivery in bone tissue engineering: progress and prospects using viral and nonviral strategies. Tissue Eng 2004;10(1–2):295–307.

21. Oligino TJ, Yao Q, Ghivizzani SC, et al. Vector systems for gene transfer to joints. Clin Orthop Relat Res 2000;379(Suppl):S17–30.

22. Wolff JA. Naked DNA transport and expression in mammalian cells. Neuromuscul Disord 1997;7(5):314–8.

23. Templeton NS, Lasic DD. New directions in liposome gene delivery. Mol Biotechnol 1999;11(2):175–80.

24. Franceschi RT, Wang D, Krebsbach PH, et al. Gene therapy for bone formation: in vitro and in vivo osteogenic activity of an adenovirus expressing BMP7. J Cell Biochem 2000;78(3):476–86.

25. Bonadio J. Tissue engineering via local gene delivery. J Mol Med 2000;78(6): 303–11.
26. Bonadio J, Smiley E, Patil P, et al. Localized, direct plasmid gene delivery in vivo: prolonged therapy results in reproducible tissue regeneration. Nat Med 1999; 5(7):753–9.
27. Shea LD, Smiley E, Bonadio J, et al. DNA delivery from polymer matrices for tissue engineering. Nat Biotechnol 1999;17(6):551–4.
28. Ramseier CA, Abramson ZR, Jin Q, et al. Gene therapeutics for periodontal regenerative medicine. Dent Clin North Am 2006;50(2):245–63, ix.
29. Giannobile WV, Lee CS, Tomala MP, et al. Platelet-derived growth factor (PDGF) gene delivery for application in periodontal tissue engineering. J Periodontol 2001;72(6):815–23.
30. Zhu Z, Lee CS, Tejeda KM, et al. Gene transfer and expression of platelet-derived growth factors modulate periodontal cellular activity. J Dent Res 2001;80(3): 892–7.
31. Anusaksathien O, Webb SA, Jin QM, et al. Platelet-derived growth factor gene delivery stimulates ex vivo gingival repair. Tissue Eng 2003;9(4):745–56.
32. Jin Q, Anusaksathien O, Webb SA, et al. Engineering of tooth-supporting structures by delivery of PDGF gene therapy vectors. Mol Ther 2004;9(4):519–26.
33. Jin QM, Anusaksathien O, Webb SA, et al. Gene therapy of bone morphogenetic protein for periodontal tissue engineering. J Periodontol 2003;74(2):202–13.
34. Lieberman JR, Daluiski A, Stevenson S, et al. The effect of regional gene therapy with bone morphogenetic protein-2-producing bone-marrow cells on the repair of segmental femoral defects in rats. J Bone Joint Surg Am 1999;81(7):905–17.
35. Baltzer AW, Lattermann C, Whalen JD, et al. Genetic enhancement of fracture repair: healing of an experimental segmental defect by adenoviral transfer of the BMP-2 gene. Gene Ther 2000;7(9):734–9.
36. Cheng SL, Lou J, Wright NM, et al. In vitro and in vivo induction of bone formation using a recombinant adenoviral vector carrying the human BMP-2 gene. Calcif Tissue Int 2001;68(2):87–94.
37. Lee JY, Musgrave D, Pelinkovic D, et al. Effect of bone morphogenetic protein-2-expressing muscle-derived cells on healing of critical-sized bone defects in mice. J Bone Joint Surg Am 2001;83-A(7):1032–9.
38. Musgrave DS, Bosch P, Ghivizzani S, et al. Adenovirus-mediated direct gene therapy with bone morphogenetic protein-2 produces bone. Bone 1999;24(6): 541–7.
39. Koh JT, Zhao Z, Wang Z, et al. Combinatorial gene therapy with BMP2/7 enhances cranial bone regeneration. J Dent Res 2008;87(9):845–9.
40. Edwards PC, Ruggiero S, Fantasia J, et al. Sonic hedgehog gene-enhanced tissue engineering for bone regeneration. Gene Ther 2005;12(1):75–86.
41. Lee JY, Peng H, Usas A, et al. Enhancement of bone healing based on ex vivo gene therapy using human muscle-derived cells expressing bone morphogenetic protein 2. Hum Gene Ther 2002;13(10):1201–11.
42. Berry M, Gonzalez AM, Clarke W, et al. Sustained effects of gene-activated matrices after CNS injury. Mol Cell Neurosci 2001;17(4):706–16.
43. Geiger F, Bertram H, Berger I, et al. Vascular endothelial growth factor gene-activated matrix (VEGF165-GAM) enhances osteogenesis and angiogenesis in large segmental bone defects. J Bone Miner Res 2005;20(11):2028–35.
44. Guo T, Zeng X, Hong H, et al. Gene-activated matrices for cartilage defect reparation. Int J Artif Organs 2006;29(6):612–21.

45. Endo M, Kuroda S, Kondo H, et al. Bone regeneration by modified gene-activated matrix: effectiveness in segmental tibial defects in rats. Tissue Eng 2006;12(3): 489–97.
46. Termaat MF, Den Boer FC, Bakker FC, et al. Bone morphogenetic proteins: development and clinical efficacy in the treatment of fractures and bone defects. J Bone Joint Surg Am 2005;87(6):1367–78.
47. Wilson JM. Medicine: a history lesson for stem cells. Science 2009;324(5928): 727–8.
48. Lin NH, Gronthos S, Bartold PM. Stem cells and periodontal regeneration. Aust Dent J 2008;53(2):108–21.
49. Thomson JA, Itskovitz-Eldor J, Shapiro SS, et al. Embryonic stem cell lines derived from human blastocysts. Science 1998;282(5391):1145–7.
50. Mitjavila-Garcia MT, Simonin C, Peschanski M. Embryonic stem cells: meeting the needs for cell therapy. Adv Drug Deliv Rev 2005;57(13):1935–43.
51. Baum CM, Weissman IL, Tsukamoto AS, et al. Isolation of a candidate human hematopoietic stem-cell population. Proc Natl Acad Sci U S A 1992;89(7):2804–8.
52. Slack JM. Stem cells in epithelial tissues. Science 2000;287(5457):1431–3.
53. Uchida N, Buck DW, He D, et al. Direct isolation of human central nervous system stem cells. Proc Natl Acad Sci U S A 2000;97(26):14720–5.
54. Castro-Malaspina H, Gay RE, Resnick G, et al. Characterization of human bone marrow fibroblast colony-forming cells (CFU-F) and their progeny. Blood 1980; 56(2):289–301.
55. Campagnoli C, Roberts IA, Kumar S, et al. Identification of mesenchymal stem/ progenitor cells in human first-trimester fetal blood, liver, and bone marrow. Blood 2001;98(8):2396–402.
56. van Imhoff GW, van der Holt B, Mackenzie MA, et al. Short intensive sequential therapy followed by autologous stem cell transplantation in adult Burkitt, Burkitt-like and lymphoblastic lymphoma. Leukemia 2005;19(6):945–52.
57. Song KW, Barnett MJ, Gascoyne RD, et al. Haematopoietic stem cell transplantation as primary therapy of sporadic adult Burkitt lymphoma. Br J Haematol 2006;133(6):634–7.
58. Bruder SP, Kurth AA, Shea M, et al. Bone regeneration by implantation of purified, culture-expanded human mesenchymal stem cells. J Orthop Res 1998;16(2): 155–62.
59. Mankani MH, Kuznetsov SA, Shannon B, et al. Canine cranial reconstruction using autologous bone marrow stromal cells. Am J Pathol 2006;168(2):542–50.
60. Kon E, Muraglia A, Corsi A, et al. Autologous bone marrow stromal cells loaded onto porous hydroxyapatite ceramic accelerate bone repair in critical-size defects of sheep long bones. J Biomed Mater Res 2000;49(3):328–37.
61. Robey PG, Kuznetsov SA, Riminucci M, et al. Skeletal (mesenchymal) stem cells for tissue engineering. Methods Mol Med 2007;140:83–99.
62. Bianco P, Robey PG. Stem cells in tissue engineering. Nature 2001;414(6859): 118–21.
63. Gurdon JB, Melton DA. Nuclear reprogramming in cells. Science 2008; 322(5909):1811–5.
64. Wilmut I, Beaujean N, de Sousa PA, et al. Somatic cell nuclear transfer. Nature 2002;419(6907):583–6.
65. Takahashi K, Yamanaka S. Induction of pluripotent stem cells from mouse embryonic and adult fibroblast cultures by defined factors. Cell 2006;126(4):663–76.
66. Yamanaka S. A fresh look at iPS cells. Cell 2009;137(1):13–7.

67. Kim JB, et al. Oct4-induced pluripotency in adult neural stem cells. Cell 2009; 136(3):411–9.
68. Yu J, Hu K, Smuga-Otto K, et al. Human induced pluripotent stem cells free of vector and transgene sequences. Science 2009;324(5928):797–801.
69. Okita K, Nakagawa M, Hyenjong H, et al. Generation of mouse induced pluripotent stem cells without viral vectors. Science 2008;322(5903):949–53.
70. Huangfu D, Osafune K, Maehr R, et al. Induction of pluripotent stem cells from primary human fibroblasts with only Oct4 and Sox2. Nat Biotechnol 2008; 26(11):1269–75.
71. Shi Y, Desponts C, Do JT, et al. Induction of pluripotent stem cells from mouse embryonic fibroblasts by Oct4 and Klf4 with small-molecule compounds. Cell Stem Cell 2008;3(5):568–74.
72. Weintraub H, Tapscott SJ, Davis RL, et al. Activation of muscle-specific genes in pigment, nerve, fat, liver, and fibroblast cell lines by forced expression of MyoD. Proc Natl Acad Sci U S A 1989;86(14):5434–8.
73. Zhou Q, Brown J, Kanarek A, et al. In vivo reprogramming of adult pancreatic exocrine cells to beta-cells. Nature 2008;455(7213):627–32.
74. Gould TR, Melcher AH, Brunette DM. Migration and division of progenitor cell populations in periodontal ligament after wounding. J Periodontal Res 1980; 15(1):20–42.
75. Isaka J, Ohazama A, Kobayashi M, et al. Participation of periodontal ligament cells with regeneration of alveolar bone. J Periodontol 2001;72(3):314–23.
76. McCulloch CA, Bordin S. Role of fibroblast subpopulations in periodontal physiology and pathology. J Periodontal Res 1991;26(3 Pt 1):144–54.
77. Seo BM, Miura M, Gronthos S, et al. Investigation of multipotent postnatal stem cells from human periodontal ligament. Lancet 2004;364(9429):149–55.
78. Gronthos S, Mrozik K, Shi S, et al. Ovine periodontal ligament stem cells: isolation, characterization, and differentiation potential. Calcif Tissue Int 2006;79(5): 310–7.
79. Shi S, Bartold PM, Miura M, et al. The efficacy of mesenchymal stem cells to regenerate and repair dental structures. Orthod Craniofac Res 2005;8(3):191–9.
80. Chen SC, Marino V, Gronthos S, et al. Location of putative stem cells in human periodontal ligament. J Periodontal Res 2006;41(6):547–53.
81. Lin NH, Menicanin D, Mrozik K, et al. Putative stem cells in regenerating human periodontium. J Periodontal Res 2008;43(5):514–23.
82. Robey PG, Bianco P. The use of adult stem cells in rebuilding the human face. J Am Dent Assoc 2006;137(7):961–72.
83. Flores MG, Hasegawa M, Yamato M, et al. Cementum-periodontal ligament complex regeneration using the cell sheet technique. J Periodontal Res 2008; 43(3):364–71.
84. Nakahara T, Nakamura T, Kobayashi E, et al. In situ tissue engineering of periodontal tissues by seeding with periodontal ligament-derived cells. Tissue Eng 2004;10(3–4):537–44.
85. Yang Z, Jin F, Zhang X, et al. Tissue engineering of cementum/periodontal-ligament complex using a novel three-dimensional pellet cultivation system for human periodontal ligament stem cells. Tissue Eng Part C Methods 2009; PMID: 19534606 [Epub ahead of print].
86. Yamada Y, Ueda M, Hibi H, et al. A novel approach to periodontal tissue regeneration with mesenchymal stem cells and platelet-rich plasma using tissue engineering technology: a clinical case report. Int J Periodontics Restorative Dent 2006;26(4):363–9.

87. Kitoh H, Kitakoji T, Tsuchiya H, et al. Transplantation of culture expanded bone marrow cells and platelet rich plasma in distraction osteogenesis of the long bones. Bone 2007;40(2):522–8.
88. Fire A, Xu S, Montgomery MK, et al. Potent and specific genetic interference by double-stranded RNA in *Caenorhabditis elegans*. Nature 1998;391(6669): 806–11.
89. Castanotto D, Rossi JJ. The promises and pitfalls of RNA-interference-based therapeutics. Nature 2009;457(7228):426–33.
90. Elbashir SM, Harborth J, Lendeckel W, et al. Duplexes of 21-nucleotide RNAs mediate RNA interference in cultured mammalian cells. Nature 2001;411(6836): 494–8.
91. Mocellin S, Provenzano M. RNA interference: learning gene knock-down from cell physiology. J Transl Med 2004;2(1):39.
92. Shen J, Samul R, Silva RL, et al. Suppression of ocular neovascularization with siRNA targeting VEGF receptor 1. Gene Ther 2006;13(3):225–34.
93. Mocellin S, Costa R, Nitti D. RNA interference: ready to silence cancer? J Mol Med 2006;84(1):4–15.
94. Li SD, Chonoc S, Huang L. Efficient oncogene silencing and metastasis inhibition via systemic delivery of siRNA. Mol Ther 2008;16(5):942–6.
95. Natarajan R, Salloum FN, Fisher BJ, et al. Hypoxia inducible factor-1 activation by prolyl 4-hydroxylase-2 gene silencing attenuates myocardial ischemia reperfusion injury. Circ Res 2006;98(1):133–40.
96. Chen LX, Lin L, Wang HJ, et al. Suppression of early experimental osteoarthritis by in vivo delivery of the adenoviral vector-mediated NF-kappaBp65-specific siRNA. Osteoarthritis Cartilage 2008;16(2):174–84.
97. Zwicky R, Müntener K, Goldring MB, et al. Cathepsin B expression and down-regulation by gene silencing and antisense DNA in human chondrocytes. Biochem J 2002;367(Pt 1):209–17.
98. Dong L, Wang R, Zhu YA, et al. Antisense oligonucleotide targeting TNF-alpha can suppress Co-Cr-Mo particle-induced osteolysis. J Orthop Res 2008;26(8): 1114–20.
99. Gazzerro E, Smerdel-Ramoya A, Zanotti S, et al. Conditional deletion of gremlin causes a transient increase in bone formation and bone mass. J Biol Chem 2007;282(43):31549–57.

Restorative Options for the Periodontal Patient

Sebastiano Andreana, DDS, MS

KEYWORDS

• Restorative dentistry • Dental implants
• All-ceramic restorations • Periodontal prosthesis

Periodontal and restorative dentistry are mutually important facets of clinical dentistry. Spear and Cooney[1] well describe the intimate relationship of these facets by stating that, "...for restorations to survive long term, the periodontium must remain healthy... for the periodontium to remain healthy, restorations must be critically managed ...so that they are in harmony with their surrounding periodontal tissues." This article discusses new techniques and trends that mostly involve this second aspect, which is the critical management of the restorations, particularly at the gingival margins. The role of implant dentistry as an option for the restorative plan of the periodontal patient is explored (**Figs. 1** and **2**).

For proper understanding of the complex relationship that exists between restorative dentistry and periodontal health, two important interrelationships are addressed: (1) the placement of the margins of a restoration and their relationship to biologic width and (2) the type of dental materials used to make the restoration.

Before describing the different possibilities available to the restorative dentist, it is essential to review important features of the anatomic structures that are naturally present where the tooth enters the alveolus, the so-called biologic width. Historically, Gargiulo and colleagues[2] described this zone as the tissues that constitute the structures above the bone crest, terminating with the free gingival margin. They promulgated a rule of thumb for the clinician to follow: the tissues above the alveolar crest fill a space composed of gingival fibers, connective tissue, and junctional epithelium that measure approximately 2 mm. Whereas this value is applicable to most clinical cases, the observations that suggested this rule were derived from the study of cadaver specimens. More recently, Vacek and colleagues[3] published a histomorphometric study that examined 171 tooth surfaces from 10 human adult cadaver jaws. This study supported the data from Gargiulo and colleagues; however, it brought attention to the fact that several variations in dimension between subjects are

Department of Restorative Dentistry, University at Buffalo, School of Dental Medicine, Buffalo, NY 14214, USA
E-mail address: andrean@buffalo.edu

Dent Clin N Am 54 (2010) 157–161
doi:10.1016/j.cden.2009.10.001
0011-8532/09/$ – see front matter © 2010 Elsevier Inc. All rights reserved.

dental.theclinics.com

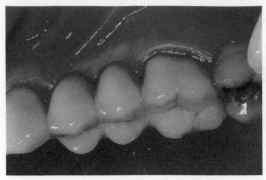

Fig. 1. Metal-ceramic crown on tooth #3. Note the fluted and flat margins at the level of the buccal furcation.

possible.[4] These investigators presented data showing large variations between subjects and, even, within the same person, with some individuals having an average biologic width of 0.75 mm and others of 4.3 mm. These variations were seen mostly within the epithelial attachment, with the connective tissue attachment having the least variability. These findings were also suggested by Gargiulo and colleagues.[2] Thus, it should be concluded that changes within the biologic width depend on the location of the tooth in the dental arch and on the individual subject. Ultimately, the 2.00 mm rule of thumb should be used with caution and interpreted on a case-by-case, tooth-by-tooth basis.

The 2.00 mm of biologic width rule has particularly influenced surgical crown lengthening procedures. The study by Landing and colleagues[5] examined the dimensions of the biologic width before and 3 and 6 months following surgical crown lengthening. Prosthetic treatment started 6 weeks after surgery. The presurgical values of biologic width were found to be reestablished 6 months after completion of the surgical procedures.

To maintain periodontal health, placing the margin of a restoration in the gingival area of the tooth is of critical importance, and violating the biologic width may lead to problems. When correlating biologic width to periodontal health and restorative margins, de Waal and Castellucci[6] suggested that the margin of the final prosthesis

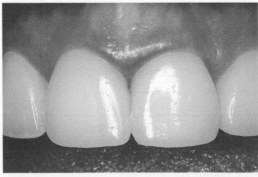

Fig. 2. Subgingival margins of all-ceramic restorations on teeth #7, #8, #9, and #10. Note gingival health.

should be placed 1 to 2 mm supragingivally wherever possible. If required for aesthetic considerations, the margin can be placed at the gingival crest or, at most, 0.25 mm to 0.5 mm into the gingival sulcus. This ensures that the biologic width remains healthy. Therefore, locating the margins of a restoration too close to the bone may cause periodontal destruction, most likely by preventing thorough plaque removal by routine oral hygiene procedures.

When the biologic width is violated, Maynard and Wilson[7] showed that an inflammatory response results in alveolar bone resorption. Furthermore, this circumstance creates a vicious circle, which leads to increased pocket depths, increased loss of periodontal support, exacerbation of accumulation of subgingival bacteria, increased chronic inflammation, and further localized periodontal breakdown.

To allow the patient the ability to maintain periodontal health, consideration should also be given to the type of crown contour that is used when fabricating the restoration. Becker and Kaldahl[8] reported that the crown contours, together with margin placement and pontic design, affect periodontal health. They suggest that the crown contour should facilitate home-care oral hygiene maneuvers, and caution that overcontoured crowns lead to increased periodontal inflammation. Their study summarizes four critical points that should be taken into account when creating crown contours: (1) buccal and lingual contours should be "flat, not fat"; (2) embrasures should be kept open; (3) the location of contact areas should be oriented toward the incisal and the buccal aspects of the restored tooth; and (4) the crown margins over furcation areas in molars and premolars should be fluted or barreled out.

Restoring molars with periodontal furcation involvement is important when attempting to preserve teeth with compromised prognosis. A recent study by Zafiropoulos and colleagues[9] evaluated the long-term outcome of hemisected mandibular molars versus teeth replaced with implants. In a group of 32 patients, 56 hemisections were performed and compared with a group of 28 patients that received 36 implants that replaced mandibular molars. All patients were categorized as having a history of chronic periodontitis, with a minimum of four sites showing attachment loss of greater than 4.00 mm, bleeding on probing of at least four sites, and radiographic evidence of bone loss. The results reported that in periodontitis patients, hemisected molars were more susceptible to complications than implants, with 32% of the hemisected teeth having some level of complications versus 11% in the implant cases.

Park and colleagues[10] reported similar findings, with 691 hemisected molars in 579 patients showing a 30% failure rate over 10 years. Periodontal complications, tooth fractures, endodontic problems, and dental caries were factors contributing to the failures. It is thus conceivable that implants are more predictable to restore and maintain masticatory function in periodontal patients than is retention of selected compromised natural teeth.

In this regard, despite the long-term success rate of implant therapy,[11-14] periodontal patients are still most often treated with conventional restorative dentistry. In the past 20 years, the dental industry has allowed the dentist to use more aesthetically pleasing materials for crown fabrication, and these new materials have demonstrated excellent results with respect to periodontal tissue tolerance. The study of Goodson and colleagues[15] conducted on nine subjects who received 42 restorations with margins made of composite gold alloys is instructive in this regard. Microbiological sampling of the crown margins were compared with samples from contralateral normal teeth. The data showed that the margins restored with porcelain/composite gold alloy had significantly fewer bacteria than contralateral normal teeth. Patients in this study were periodontally healthy. Subsequently, in 2002, a study by Gemalnaz and Ergin[16] was conducted on 37 all-ceramic crowns placed in 20 patients. Among other restorative parameters, plaque and gingival scores were also assessed for a period averaging 25 months after cementation. Incisors, premolars, and molars were included in this study. The all-ceramic crowns showed significantly less plaque growth than did natural teeth. Differences in favor of the artificial crowns were also reported when assessing gingival inflammation. When location of margins was considered, subgingival margins were more prone to have bleeding on probing than were supragingival margins. The study by Felton and colleagues[17] of 29 patients indicated that marginal discrepancies were associated with gingival inflammation. An accurate impression technique is always required to reduce subgingival microgaps between the restorative margins and the tooth preparation margins and, therefore, minimize plaque formation.

SUMMARY

Periodontal health and restorative dentistry are inextricably linked. Today's clinicians have many treatment options at their disposal, including biotolerant restorative materials and implants, to maintain periodontal health. Nevertheless, it is crucial for the clinician to understand the biologic principles that form the foundation for restorative reconstruction of the periodontally involved tooth.

REFERENCES

1. Spear FM, Cooney JP. Restorative interrelationships. In: Newman MG, Takei HH, Klokkevold PR, et al, editors. Carranza's Clinical Periodontology. Tenth edition. Philadelphia: Saunders Elsevier; 2006. Chapter 72. p. 1050–69.
2. Gargiulo AW, Wentz FM, Orban B. Dimensions and relations of the dentogingival junction in humans. J Periodontol 1961;32:261–7.
3. Vacek JS, Gher ME, Assad DA, et al. The dimensions of the human dentogingival junction. Int J Periodontics Restorative Dent 1994;14(2):154–65.
4. Andreana S. Understanding the biologic width: a practical approach. Pract Proced Aesthet Dent 2007;19(6):374–6.
5. Landing SK, Waldrop TC, Gunsolley JC, et al. Surgical crown lengthening: evaluation of the biological width. J Periodontol 2003;74(4):468–74.
6. de Waal H, Castellucci G. The importance of restorative margin placement to the biologic width and periodontal health. Part II. Int J Periodontics Restorative Dent 1994;14(1):70–83.
7. Maynard JG Jr, Wilson RD. Physiologic dimensions of the periodontium significant to the restorative dentist. J Periodontol 1979;50(4):170–4.
8. Becker CM, Kaldahl WB. Current theories of crown contour, margin placement, and pontic design 1981. J Prosthet Dent 2005;93(2):107–15.
9. Zafiropoulos GG, Hoffmann O, Kasaj A, et al. Mandibular molar root resection versus implant therapy: a retrospective nonrandomized study. J Oral Implantol 2009;35(2):52–62.
10. Park SY, Shin SY, Yang SM, et al. Factors influencing the outcome of root-resection therapy in molars: a 10-year retrospective study. J Periodontol 2009;80(1):32–40.
11. van Steenberghe D, Lekholm U, Bolender C, et al. Applicability of osseointegrated oral implants in the rehabilitation of partial edentulism: a prospective multicenter study on 558 fixtures. Int J Oral Maxillofac Implants 1990;5(3):272–81.
12. Brocard D, Barthet P, Baysse E, et al. A multicenter report on 1,022 consecutively placed ITI implants: a 7-year longitudinal study. Int J Oral Maxillofac Implants. 2000;15(5):691–700.

13. Lekholm U, Gröndahl K, Jemt T. Outcome of oral implant treatment in partially edentulous jaws followed 20 years in clinical function. Clin Implant Dent Relat Res 2006;8(4):178–86.
14. Andreana S, Beneduce C, Buhite R. Implant success rate in dental school setting: retrospective study. N Y State Dent J 2008;74(5):67–70.
15. Goodson JM, Shorer I, Imber S, et al. Reduced dental plaque accumulation on composite gold alloy margins. J Periodont Res 2001;36:252–9.
16. Gemalnaz D, Ergin S. Clinical evaluation of all-ceramic crowns. J Prosthet Dent 2002;87:189–96.
17. Felton DA, Kanoy BE, Bayne SC, et al. Effect of in vivo crown margin discrepancies on periodontal health. J Prosthet Dent 1991;65(3):357–64.

"Does Periodontal Therapy Reduce the Risk for Systemic Diseases?"

Frank A. Scannapieco, DMD, PhD[a],*,
Ananda P. Dasanayake, BDS, MPH, PhD, FACE[b], Nok Chhun, MS, MPH[c]

KEYWORDS

- Periodontal disease • Periodontal therapy • Periodontitis
- Systemic diseases

As detailed in the previous articles in this issue, periodontal disease is treated by various approaches, from simple oral hygiene practices and professional mechanical debridment, and antimicrobial therapy, to periodontal surgery that may involve the use of bone grafts, guided tissue regeneration, growth factors and beyond. Treatment is almost always rendered to manage the local effects of periodontitis, that is the localized destruction of the tooth attachment apparatus by inflammation induced by the bacteria of dental plaque.

In the past two decades evidence has emerged associating periodontal disease with several important systemic diseases and conditions. Results from numerous case-control and epidemiologic studies suggest that people with periodontal disease have a modestly higher risk for myocardial infarction (MI) when compared with people without periodontal disease. Other studies have also connected periodontal disease with adverse pregnancy outcomes,[1,2] diabetes mellitus,[3] various lung diseases such as pneumonia and chronic obstructive lung disease,[4] and Alzheimer's disease.[5] In the future, there may be additional justification for such therapy should periodontal disease be proven to influence the initiation or progression of systemic diseases such as atherosclerosis, adverse pregnancy outcomes, diabetes mellitus, or chronic lung disease.

[a] Department of Oral Biology, School of Dental Medicine, University at Buffalo, The State University of New York, Foster Hall, Buffalo, NY 14214, USA
[b] Graduate Program in Clinical Research, New York University College of Dentistry, 250 Park Avenue South - 6th Floor - Room 646, New York, NY 10003-1402, USA
[c] Graduate Program in Clinical Research, Department of Epidemiology, New York University College of Dentistry, 250 Park Avenue South - 6th Floor - Room 646, New York, NY 10003-1402, USA
* Corresponding author.
E-mail address: fas1@buffalo.edu (F.A. Scannapieco).

Dent Clin N Am 54 (2010) 163–181
doi:10.1016/j.cden.2009.10.002
0011-8532/09/$ – see front matter © 2010 Elsevier Inc. All rights reserved.

What is the evidence for the efficacy of periodontal therapy in the treatment or prevention of systemic disease? A complete review of the literature that addresses all evidence for or against a role for periodontal disease in the pathogenesis of systemic diseases is beyond the scope of the present article. Instead, the published literature that describes the effects of periodontal treatment on cardiovascular diseases (CVDs), adverse pregnancy outcomes, diabetes mellitus, and respiratory disease is reviewed.

CVD

Although it is unknown how periodontal disease influences the course of atherosclerosis, several mechanisms have been proposed involving direct effects of periodontal bacteria that injure vascular tissue, and indirect effects mediated through innate and specific immune responses against periodontal bacteria causing vasculature damage.[6] Regardless of mechanism, it has been assumed that periodontal treatment would reduce the insult imposed by the microorganisms of dental plaque to reduce the inflammatory response and thus atherosclerosis.

In July 2009 a computer search using the following search terms was conducted using PubMed: periodontal; treatment; cardiovascular; randomized; and trial. A total of twenty one articles were retrieved. Although no studies have been published that measure the effect of periodontal treatment on a clinical outcome such as MI, seven papers were chosen for review that describe a well-designed randomized trial that measured surrogate markers believed to serve as risk indicators for MI. Risk indicators measured included acute-phase response markers such as C-reactive protein (CRP), fibrinogen, serum α-amyloid A, and proinflammatory cytokines such as interleukin 1β (IL-1β), IL-6, and tumor necrosis factor α (TNF-α) (**Table 1**). In some cases, flow-mediated vascular dilatation was measured.[9,11,12]

Although most of these trials showed reduction in one or more surrogate markers for atherosclerosis activity following periodontal therapy,[8–12] several trials showed no effect.[7,15]

Most of these trials are small, enrolling between 30 and 65 patients, with the exception of the study of Tonetti and colleagues,[12] which enrolled 120 patients, and the Periodontal and Vascular Events (PAVE) study, which enrolled 303 patients.[13] Typically, the active treatment involved professional mechanical debridment compared with a control group that received the treatment at the end of the trial after measurement of outcomes. Treatment sometimes included periodontal surgery or systemic or local administration of antibiotics. In some cases the control group were untreated periodontal patients, or patients who received community care versus purposeful intervention by a study investigator.

The available results must be interpreted with caution. The lack of an accepted standard for treatment of periodontitis presents considerable heterogeneity in results. Variations in treatment (eg, scaling and root planing (SRP) alone, with or without surgery, with or without antibiotics) yield results that may be difficult to interpret. Should patients receive only one course of local debridment, or should they be treated until they demonstrate an absence of periodontal inflammation? These different periodontal end points would greatly modify study design and the cost and duration of a clinical trial. The sample size of most of the studies may be underpowered to detect all but robust treatment effects. Because the primary outcome of interest (MI) is of low prevalence in most populations, large sample sizes are required to detect differences in treatment arms should such differences exist. Such studies are expensive to run. The length of trials may be too brief in duration to observe meaningful outcomes.

Indeed, clinical outcomes of processes such as atherosclerosis (eg, MI) are often years in the making. Perhaps a short-term periodontal treatment might not have a discernable effect on such long-term clinical outcomes.

ADVERSE PREGNANCY OUTCOMES

Periodontal disease is related to increased inflammatory mediators and prostaglandins and some of these molecules such as prostaglandin E_2 (PGE_2) are known to influence preterm delivery.[2] In this regard, it is possible that pregnant women with periodontal disease experience more preterm deliveries. Before evaluating the results of periodontal disease treatment trials in relation to poor pregnancy outcomes, it is useful to understand the existing body of literature that links periodontal disease with poor pregnancy outcomes. To establish such an association using observational studies, clinical, bacteriologic, immunologic, and inflammatory mediator outcomes related to periodontal disease must be measured without any errors and their independent effect on poor pregnancy outcomes should be measured, using either a prospective, case-control, or cross-sectional studies with adequate numbers of subjects, while taking into account potential confounding factors.[2] Measurement of elements related to periodontal disease locally and systemically, and specifically within the fetoplacental unit, and within a time period that makes biologic sense in relation to pregnancy outcomes, would validate observational studies. As of October, 2009, 88 studies from populations around the world have been published that address the potential link between parameters related to periodontal disease and poor pregnancy outcomes such as low birth weight, preterm birth, and preterm low birth weight. These studies, their location, the periodontal parameters that were evaluated, and the nature of the association of these parameters with poor pregnancy outcomes (positive association [+] or no association [−]) are depicted in **Fig. 1**. Fifty of these studies reported a significant association, although 24 studies failed to find an association.

Such a depiction, however, does not take into account the inherent strengths or the limitations of these studies. One way to evaluate the association between periodontal disease and pregnancy outcomes is to pool the results from these studies, while taking into account their strengths and weaknesses. Meta-analysis of existing studies allows this to some extent. Based on 17 observational studies, Vergnes and Sixou[14] concluded that the overall association between periodontal disease and preterm low birth weight was statistically significant (overall odds ratio [OR] = 2.83; 95% confidence interval [CI] = 1.95–4.10). However, this may not be accurate either as some studies suffer from residual confounding caused by inadequately controlled factors such as smoking. One way to remove this "threat" is to conduct a study within a population in which pregnant women do not engage in risk behaviors such as smoking, alcohol consumption, and drug use. As these behaviors are causally related to poor pregnancy outcomes and are also related to periodontal disease, by removing the effect of such factors from the association between periodontal disease and poor pregnancy outcomes, the credibility of this association can be enhanced. By studying Sri Lankan women who do not engage in these behaviors because of economic and cultural barriers, in a prospective study it has been reported that the unconfounded association between clinical periodontal disease and preterm delivery is not statistically significant.[15]

Definitive evidence to test this association, however, could come from large randomized clinical trials, as they are generally not subjected to the limitations of observational studies discussed earlier. By randomly allocating sufficient numbers of patients to treatment and control groups, a better control of potential confounding factors and biases can be achieved. However, the results from randomized trials are

Table 1

Intervention studies of periodontal treatment to improve periodontal status and reduce surrogate markers of CVD risk.

Citations	Number of Subjects (Placebo/Control)	Treatment	Outcomes Measured	Results	Comments
Ide et al[7]	39 nonsmoking subjects with moderate to advanced chronic periodontitis. Random assignment to immediate treatment or treatment following a 3-month non-treatment phase	Full-mouth scaling and root planing	Dental outcomes: plaque index, bleeding on probing, pocket depths. CVD outcomes: serum levels of CRP, fibrinogen, serum α-amyloid A, IL-1β, IL-6, and TNF-α	Treatment significantly improved periodontal status. No significant changes in levels of any of the systemic markers were noted	Small number of patients examined
D'Aiuto et al[8]	40 systemically healthy subjects with severe generalized chronic periodontitis. Random assignment to either standard treatment (20 subjects) or intensive treatment (20 subjects) and followed for 6-month trial	SPT: only full-mouth scaling and root planing of all teeth. IPT: full-mouth scaling and root planing of all teeth plus adjunctive local delivery of minocycline microspheres (Arestin, OraPharma, Warminster, PA)	Dental outcomes: average full-mouth supragingival plaque scores, average full-mouth gingival bleeding scores, and average full-mouth number of periodontal lesions. CVD outcomes: serum CRP, IL-6, leukocyte counts, HDL-C, BP, body mass index, Framingham risk scores	Both treatments improved periodontal status compared with baseline. IPT showed significant reductions in inflammatory markers (IL-6 and CRP) and lipid markers (TC and LDL-C) at 2 and 6 months, no changes were observed for systemic markers in the SPT group. Both treatments reduced leukocyte counts at 6 months. BP reduced after 2 months by IPT.	Small number of patients examined; all subjects had severe, generalized periodontitis

| Mercanoglu et al[9] | 54 subjects were enrolled - 28 with chronic periodontitis and without atherosclerotic disease, and 26 healthy controls. Subjects with periodontitis were compared with subjects with healthy periodontium; all subjects received the same treatment | Scaling and root planning of all teeth | Dental outcomes: PI, GI, PD, and CAL, radiographic bone levels. CVD outcomes: flow-mediated dilatation of the brachial artery following transient ischemia | Periodontal therapy significantly reduced mean PI, GI, PD, and CAL of the periodontitis group. Increases in brachial artery diameter induced by reactive hyperemia and sublingual nitroglycerine in the periodontitis group were significantly less than the control group at baseline. There was no significant difference between the initial and final measurements of flow-mediated dilatation in the control subjects. After periodontal treatment, the changes in brachial artery diameter induced by reactive hyperemia and sublingual nitroglycerine in the posttreatment measurements were significantly higher when compared with initial measurements | Endothelial functions in patients with chronic periodontitis were impaired compared with subjects without periodontitis. Recovery of endothelial dysfunction after periodontal treatment was demonstrated. Small number of patients examined. |

(continued on next page)

Table 1 *(continued)*

Citations	Number of Subjects (Placebo/Control)	Treatment	Outcomes Measured	Results	Comments
D'Aiuto et al[10]	65 subjects with severe periodontitis. Random assignment to untreated control group (24 subjects); standard periodontal treatment group (SPT: 21 subjects), or an intensive periodontal treatment (IPT: 20 subjects), consisting of SPT plus local minocycline hydrochloride for 2 months	SPT: only full-mouth scaling and root planing of all teeth. IPT: full-mouth scaling and root planing of all teeth plus adjunctive local delivery of minocycline microspheres (Arestin, OraPharma, Warminster, PA)	Dental outcomes: percentage of tooth sites with dental plaque, percentage of tooth sites with bleeding on probing, full-mouth average periodontal pocket depth, full-mouth average clinical attachment loss. CVD outcomes: CRP, IL-6, total cholesterol, and LDL-C	Periodontal therapy (either standard or intensive) resulted in an additional reduction in serum CRP of at least 0.5 mg/L compared with the untreated controls	SPT and IPT resulted in statistically significant reductions of periodontal lesions after therapy. No changes were observed in the untreated controls
Seinost et al[11]	30 patients with severe periodontitis and 31 control subjects were assessed FMD of the brachial artery	All patients received oral hygiene instructions, scaling and root planing of all teeth. CHX (0.1%) mouth rinses for 14 days, and systemic amoxicillin plus clavulanic acid and metronidazole therapy was administered for 7 days. Residual pockets of more than 5 mm that bled after probing were rescaled 12 weeks after periodontal treatment	Dental outcomes: bleeding on probing, probing depth, gingival recession. CVD outcomes: measurement of serum total cholesterol, triglycerides, HDL, Hb A$_{1c}$, LDL-C, CRP. Brachial artery reactivity was assessed within 1 week of the initial treatment and 3 months after end of treatment	Subjects with periodontitis had significantly higher baseline levels CRP than controls. After periodontal treatment, CRP significantly decreased. FMD expressed as change in diameter and as percent change was significantly lower in patients with periodontitis before treatment than in healthy controls after 3 months. Nitroglycerin-associated dilation did not differ significantly between controls and patients with periodontitis before and after treatment	

Tonetti et al[12]	120 patients with severe periodontitis. Random assignment of 59 subjects to community-based periodontal care/61 to intensive periodontal treatment followed for 6 months	Full-mouth scaling and root planing; extraction of hopeless teeth; local placement of microspheres of minocycline into periodontal pockets	Dental outcomes: dental plaque score, gingival bleeding on probing score, periodontal pocket depth, gingival recession, CVD outcomes: endothelial function by FMD of the brachial artery, serum CRP, IL-6, soluble E-selectin, t-PA, PAI-1, and von Willebrand factor	Significantly greater FMD in the treatment group compared with control-treatment after 60 days. Plasma levels of soluble E-selectin were lower in the intensive-treatment group than in the control group	
Offenbacher et al[13]	303 subjects with periodontal disease and a history of blockage of 1 coronary artery or, a coronary artery event, including MI, coronary artery bypass graft surgery, or coronary transluminal angioplasty with or without a stent. Random assignment of 152 subjects to community-based periodontal care/151 to periodontal treatment	Full-mouth scaling and root planing	Dental outcomes: periodontal probing depth, bleeding on probing, and periodontal attachment level, GCF IL-1β. CVD outcomes: serum hs-CRP	Improved periodontal status in treatment group (pocket reduction). No reduction in GCF IL-1β or serum hs-CRP concentrations in treatment group compared with community controls	Obesity and periodontal treatment in some community controls may have confounded data interpretation

Abbreviations: BP, blood pressure; CAL, clinical attachment level; FMD, flow-mediated dilation; GCF, gingival crevicular fluid; GI, gingival index; HDL-C, high-density lipoprotein cholesterol; IPT, intensive periodontal therapy; LDL-C, low-density lipoprotein cholesterol; PAI-1, plasminogen-activator inhibitor type 1; PD, probing depth; PI, plaque index; SPT, standard periodontal therapy; TC, total cholesterol; t-PA, tissue plasminogen activator.

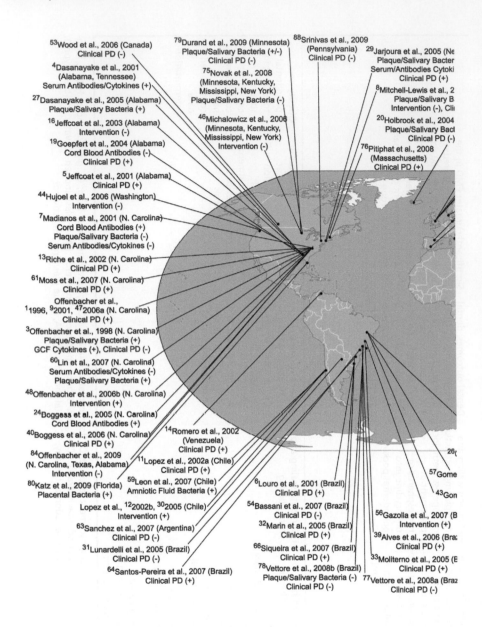

equivocal. Whereas studies conducted in Chile[16–18] suggest that periodontal treatment given to pregnant women with gingivitis or periodontitis results in a reduction of preterm low birth weight, studies conducted in the United States failed to observe similar results.[19,20] It is unlikely that this discrepancy is caused by population differences. Whereas the Chilean studies provided mechanical periodontal treatment as needed during pregnancy, the US studies were restricted to a limited number of scaling and root planning sessions. However, careful review of one of the US studies, suggests that other pregnancy outcomes such as spontaneous abortion and stillbirth were significantly reduced in the treatment group.[19] In a treatment study in which

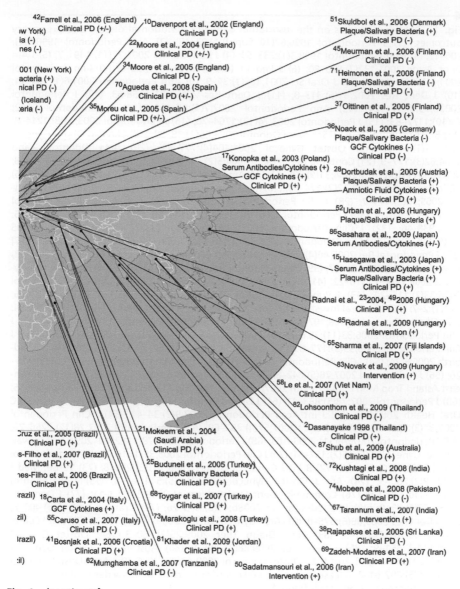

Fig. 1. *(continued)*

metronidazole was used, Jeffcoat and colleagues[21] observed an increased risk of preterm birth in the treatment group. All studies have shown that periodontal treatment rendered during pregnancy was safe.

Among the potential explanations for these discrepancies are inappropriate timing of treatment, inadequacy of treatment, and limitations in the selected outcomes. Despite these concerns, when data from seven of these randomized trials were pooled using meta-analysis, Polyzos and colleagues[22] showed that periodontal treatment during pregnancy significantly reduced preterm birth (OR = 0.55; 95% CI = 0.35–0.86) but not low birth weight (OR = 0.48, 95% CI = 0.23–1.0).

Fig. 1 . Published studies on the association between periodontal disease and pregnancy outcomes. (1) J Periodontol 1996;67(10 Suppl):1103–13; (2) Ann Periodontol 1998;3(1): 206–12; (3) Ann Periodontol 1998;3(1):233–50; (4) J Periodontol 2001;72(11):1491–7; (5) J Am Dent Assoc 2001;132(7):875–80; (6) J Pediatr (Rio J) 2001;77(1):23–8; (7) Ann Periodontol 2001;6(1):175–82; (8) Eur J Oral Sci 2001;109(1):34–9; (9) Ann Periodontol 2001;6(1):164–74; (10) J Dent Res 2002;81(5):313–8; (11) J Dent Res 2002a;81(1):58-63; (12) J Periodontol 2002b;73(8):911–24; (13) Ann Periodontol 2002;7(1):95–101; (14) J Periodontol 2002; 73(10):1177–83; (15) J Periodontol 2003;74(12):1764–70; (16) J Periodontol 2003;74(8):1214–8; (17) Bull Group Int Rech Sci Stomatol Odontol 2003;45(1):18–28; (18) Clin Exp Obstet Gynecol 2004;31(1):47–9; (19) Obstet Gynecol 2004;104(4):777–83; (20) Acta Odontol Scand 2004;62(3):177–9; (21) Contemp Dent Pract J 2004;5(2):40–56; (22) Br Dent J 2004;197(5):251–8; (23) J Clin Periodontol 2004;31(9):736–41; (24) Am J Obstet Gynecol 2005;193(3 Pt 2):1121–6; (25) J Clin Periodontol 2005;32(2):174–81; (26) Rev Saude Publica 2005;39(5):782–7; (27) J Periodontol 2005;76(2):171–7; (28) J Clin Periodontol 2005;32(1):45–52; (29) Am J Obstet Gynecol 2005;192(2):513–9; (30) J Periodontol 2005;76(11 Suppl):2144–53; (31) J Clin Periodontol 2005; 32(9):938–46; (32) J Clin Periodontol 2005;32(3):299–304; (33) J Clin Periodontol 2005 ;32(8):886–90; (34) J Clin Periodontol 2005;32(1):1–5; (35) J Clin Periodontol 2005;32(6):622–7; (36) J Periodontal Res 2005;40(4):339–45; (37) Infect Dis Obstet Gynecol 2005;13(4):213–6; (38) J Dent Res 2005;84(3):274–7; (39) Pesqui Odontol Bras 2006;20(4):318–23; (40) Am J Obstet Gynecol 2006;194(5):1316–22; (41) J Clin Periodontol 2006;33(10):710–6; (42) J Clin Periodontol 2006;33(2):115–20; (43) J Public Health Dent 2006;66(4):295–8; (44) Eur J Oral Sci 2006; 114(1):2–7; (45) Clin Oral Investig 2006;10(2):96–101; (46) N Engl J Med 2006;355(18):1885–94; (47) Obstet Gynecol 2006a;107(1):29–36; (48) J Periodontol 2006b;77(12):2011–2024; (49) J Clin Periodontol 2006;33(11):791–6; (50) J Indian Soc Pedod Prev Dent 2006;24(1):23–6; (51) J Clin Periodontol 2006;33(3):177–83; (52) Anaerobe 2006;12(1):52–7; (53) BMC Pregnancy Childbirth 2006;6:24; (54) J Clin Periodontol 2007;34(1):31–9; (55) Minerva Stomatol 2007;56(9):415–26; (56) J Periodontol 2007;78(5):842–8; (57) J Clin Periodontol 2007;34(11):957–63; (58) Southeast Asian J Trop Med Public Health 2007;38(3):586–93; (59) J Periodontol 2007;78(7):1249–55; (60) J Periodontol 2007;78(5):833–41; (61) J Oral Maxillofac Surg 2007;65(9):1739–45; (62) BMC Oral Health 2007;7:8; (63) J Int Acad Periodontol 2007;9(2):34–41; (64) J Clin Periodontol 2007;34(3):208–13; (65) Int Dent J 2007;57(4):257–60; (66) J Periodontol 2007;78(12):2266–76; (67) J Periodontol 2007;78(11):2095–103; (68) J Periodontol 2007;78(11):2081–2094; (69) Taiwan J Obstet Gynecol 2007;46(2):157–61; (70) J Clin Periodontol 2008;35(1):16–22; (71) Acta Odontol Scand 2008;66(6):334–41; (72) B Int J Gynaecol Obstet 2008;101(3):296–8; (73) Yonsei Med J 2008;49(2):200–3; (74) Am J Obstet Gynecol 2008;198(5):514 e1–8; (75) J Periodontol 2008;79(10):1870–9; (76) Community Dent Oral Epidemiol 2008;36(1):3–11; (77) J Dent Res 2008a;87(1):73–8; (78) J Periodontal Res 2008b;43(6):615–26; (79) Oral Dis 2009;15(6):400–6; (80) J Dent Res 2009;88(6):575–8; (81) Arch Gynecol Obstet 2009;279(2):165–9; (82) Am J Epidemiol 2009;169(6):731–9; (83) Fetal Diagn Ther 2009;25(2):230–3; (84) Obstet Gynecol 2009;114(3):551–9; (85) J Dent Res 2009;88(3):280–4; (86) Aust N Z J Obstet Gynaecol 2009;9(2):137–41; (87) Aust N Z J Obstet Gynaecol 2009;49(2):130–6; (88) Am J Obstet Gynecol 2009;200(5):497 e1–8. (Please see online version of this article at www.dental.theclinics.com for an enhanced version of this figure.)

In conclusion, the "jury is still out" on the role of periodontal disease in poor pregnancy outcomes. A definitive, adequately powered human experimental study is required that demonstrates a correlation between conversion of poor periodontal status to health in the treatment group for the duration of pregnancy, with a parallel reduction in adverse pregnancy outcomes. Until then, it can be concluded that periodontal treatment is safe for pregnant women, and that women should maintain good periodontal health before, during, and after pregnancy.

DIABETES

Diabetes is a metabolic disorder that is caused either by hypoproduction of insulin or improper use of available insulin that, in both cases, leads to high blood glucose levels. The American Diabetes Association estimates that there are 23.6 million children and adults (7.8%) in the United States with diabetes. Close to 6 million of these people are unaware that they have diabetes. In addition, another 57 million people are in the prediabetic stage (http://www.diabetes.org/about-diabetes.jsp). Globally, it is estimated that 4.4% of the world's population of all ages will suffer from diabetes by the year 2030.[23]

Periodontal disease is more common (60%) in people with diabetes.[24] Young adults with diabetes have about twice the risk of periodontal disease than those without diabetes. Almost one-third of people with diabetes have severe periodontal disease with loss of attachment of the gums to the teeth measuring 5 mm or more. Persons with poorly controlled diabetes (hemoglobin A_{1c}[Hb A_{1c}] > 9%) are nearly 3 times more likely to have severe periodontal disease than those without diabetes. Among the biologic mechanisms that explain why diabetes adversely affects periodontal tissues are microangiopathy, genetic predisposition, alterations in gingival crevicular fluid, collagen metabolism, host inflammatory response, and the quality of the subgingival flora.[25]

Periodontal infection may also adversely affect glycemic control. The highly vascularized and inflamed periodontium may serve as an endocrinelike source for TNF-α and other inflammatory mediators that are known to influence glucose and lipid metabolism, at least in acute circumstances. TNF-α, IL-6, and IL-1β are known insulin antagonists. As such, attempts have been made to evaluate the effect of periodontal treatment on glycemic control.

A meta-analysis of several controlled clinical trials[26,27–30] has shown that the periodontal treatment group showed a 0.8% reduction in HbA_{1c} levels (95% CI = 0.2%–1.4%).[31] However, these findings are difficult to interpret as they are based on predominantly male subjects (71%) who were in their late 50s (mean age = 58.1 years) with primarily type II diabetes (83.4%), and a higher prevalence of smoking (42.3%). Variability in periodontal treatment also makes it hard to interpret these findings. Although most subjects received SRP, some received either local or systemic antibiotics, whereas others used antiseptics. There were also differences across studies in the type of diabetes and glycemic control and the study duration. A randomized control trial that is designed to overcome these limitations is under way in Europe.[32]

GESTATIONAL DIABETES

According to the American Diabetes Association, pregnant women who have never had diabetes but who have high blood sugar (glucose) levels during pregnancy are considered to have gestational diabetes. Gestational diabetes affects about 4% of all pregnant women (about 135,000 cases of gestational diabetes) in the United States each year. Epidemiologic studies have linked periodontal disease to gestational diabetes in the United States and in other populations. Because inflammatory mediators related to periodontal disease such as TNF-α, IL-6, and IL-1 are known insulin antagonists, it is possible that pregnant women with periodontal disease have a higher risk for gestational diabetes. Several cross-sectional studies demonstrated an association between clinical periodontal disease and gestational diabetes using data from the Third National Health and Nutrition Examination Survey (NHANES III).[33,34] A subsequent case-control study[35] also found a 2.5-fold increase in gestational diabetes among pregnant women with periodontal disease (95% CI = 1.1–6.1). Although

Table 2
Published intervention studies of oral disinfection with CHX to prevent VAP.

References	Number of Subjects (Study/Placebo/Control)	Randomization	Oral Intervention	Result (Placebo vs Control)	Side Effects/ Adverse Reactions
DeRiso et al[41]	Cardiovascular ICU subjects: 173 subjects in test group, 180 subjects in placebo group. All received systemic antibiotics	Yes	0.12% CHX oral rinse (with 11.6% ethanol), 0.5 oz for 30 s, twice a day. Placebo (with ethanol 3.2%) 0.5 oz for 30 s twice a day	69% reduction in total respiratory tract infections in the CHX group (P<.05). A reduction in mortality in the CHX-group (1.16% vs 5.56%)	Not reported
Genuit et al[42]	Prospective study of 95 surgical ICU patients who required mechanical ventilation compared with 39 historic controls	No	0.12% CHX oral rinse twice a day with ventilator WP. "Placebo control" only WP	WP and CHX led to significant reduction and delay of occurrence of VAP (37% overall, 75% for late VAP, P<.05).	Not reported
Houston et al[43]	Prospective study of 270 cardiac surgical patients in test group compared with 291 in placebo group	Yes	0.12% CHX gluconate twice a day versus placebo (Listerine), both delivered twice a day for 10 days postoperatively	52% reduction in the overall rate of pneumonia in the 0.12% CHX gluconate-treated patients. A 71% reduction in the rate of pneumonia among patients intubated for more than 24 h with heavy growth in the sputum samples and treated with 0.12% CHX gluconate (2/10 vs 7/10; P = .02)	Not reported
Flanders et al[37]	Prospective study of 228 mechanically ventilated patients in the CHX group compared with 228 patients in the placebo group	Yes	0.2% CHX gel 3 times a day, during the entire ICU stay; placebo gel, 3 times a day, during the entire ICU stay	Did not reduce nosocomial infections (18.4% in the test group versus 17.5% in the control group). CHX did lower positive dental plaque cultures in the treated group versus placebo on day 10 (29% vs 66%)	No side effects were reported

Koeman et al[44]	Yes	Prospective study of 127 ICU patients treated with 2% CHX, 128 with 2% CHX plus topical colistin and 130 with placebo	CHX 2% in petroleum jelly [Vaseline], CHX 2% with COL 2% in Vaseline, and Vaseline. All applied 4 times a day to each side of the oral cavity	The daily risk of VAP was statistically significantly reduced in both treatment groups compared with placebo. CHX/COL provided significant reduction in oropharyngeal colonization with gram-negative and gram-positive microorganisms, whereas CHX mostly affected gram-positive microorganisms	One patient in the CHX/COL group was withdrawn from the trial because of tongue edema
Segers et al[45]	Yes	Prospective study of 991 patients randomly assigned to the 2 treatment groups	A 0.12% CHX solution was used as an oral rinse and as a gel for nasal application	A total of 96 patients (19.8%) in the CHX group were diagnosed with 116 nosocomial infections compared with 123 patients (26.2%) with 164 nosocomial infections in the placebo group (ARR, 6.4%; 95% CI, 1.1%–11.7%; $P = .002$)	An adverse effect from CHX was observed in 1 patient (0.2%) who experienced temporary minor discoloration of the teeth
Tantipong et al[46]	Yes	CHX group (n = 102) and normal saline group (n = 105)	2% CHX solution or normal saline solution 4 times per day until endotracheal tube was removed	The rate of VAP in the CHX group was 7 episodes per 1000 ventilator-days, and the rate in the normal saline group was 21 episodes per 1000 ventilator-days ($P = .04$)	Irritation of the oral mucosa was observed in 10 (9.8%) of the patients in the CHX group and in 1 (0.9%) of the patients in the normal saline group ($P = .001$)

(continued on next page)

Table 2
(continued)

References	Number of Subjects (Study/Placebo/Control)	Randomization	Oral Intervention	Result (Placebo vs Control)	Side Effects/Adverse Reactions
Bellissimo-Rodrigues et al[47]	194 patients admitted to the ICU with a prospective length of stay greater than 48 h	Yes	Randomized into 2 groups: 0.12% CHX (n = 98) or placebo (n = 96), applied 3 times a day throughout the duration of the patient's stay in the ICU	No difference between groups for all outcomes except time to onset of the first respiratory tract infection, in which case patients in the CHX group exhibited a longer interval between ICU admission and onset of the first respiratory tract infection than did the control patients (11.3 vs 7.6 days; P = .05)	No severe adverse events related to CHX were reported
Panchabhai et al[48]	512 patients were randomized	Yes	Twice-daily oropharyngeal cleansing with 0.2% CHX or 0.01% potassium permanganate (control) solution	Nosocomial pneumonia developed in 16 of 224 subjects (7.1%) in the CHX group and 19 of 247 subjects (7.7%) in the control group (P = 0.82; relative risk, 0.93; 95% CI, 0.49 to 1.76)	Not reported
Scannapieco et al[49]	175 subjects were randomized; microbiologic baseline data were available for 146 subjects, with 115 subjects having full outcome assessment after at least 48 h	Yes	Oral topical 0.12% CHX or placebo (vehicle alone), applied once or twice a day by staff nurses	CHX reduced the number of S aureus, but not the total number of enterics, Pseudomonas or Acinetobacter in the dental plaque of test subjects. A nonsignificant reduction in pneumonia rate was noted in groups treated with CHX compared with the placebo group	No adverse effects reported
Munro et al[50]	192 subjects admitted to medical, surgical/trauma, and neuro-ICUs with appropriate data on days 1 and 3 for analysis	Yes	Comparison of mechanical (toothbrushing), CHX, a combination (toothbrushing plus CHX), versus usual oral care for 7 days	CHX significantly reduced the incidence of pneumonia on day 3 (CPIS ≥6) among patients who had CPIS <6 at baseline (P = .006). Toothbrushing had no effect on CPIS and did not enhance the effect of CHX	Not reported

Abbreviations: ARR, absolute risk reduction; CHX, chlorhexidine gluconate; COL, colistin; CPIS, clinical pulmonary infection score; VAP, ventilator associated pneumonia; WP, weaning protocol.

cross-sectional and case-control studies cannot address the temporal sequence of the association, a recent longitudinal study reported that periodontal pathogens in vaginal samples were significantly associated with gestational diabetes.[2] By selecting a homogenous group of Asian women who are at high risk for gestational diabetes, it was observed that a statistically significant association existed between bleeding on probing and higher glucose challenge test values among nonsmoking Sri Lankan women after controlling for age (OR = 3.5; 95% = 1.2–10.4).[36] However, there are no studies addressing the effect of periodontal treatment during pregnancy on gestational diabetes.

PNEUMONIA

Pneumonia is characterized by inflammation of the lungs resulting from infection with bacteria, viruses, and other microorganisms. Hospital-acquired pneumonia (HAP), defined as pneumonia with an onset 48 hours or more after admission to the hospital, is a common and costly nosocomial infection, causing considerable morbidity and mortality.[37] Ventilator-associated pneumonia (VAP), a subset of HAP, is defined as pneumonia developing 48 hours or more after initiation of mechanical ventilation.[38] The pathogenesis of pneumonia depends on the aspiration of bacteria from the oral cavity and upper airway into the lungs, and subsequent failure of host defenses to clear the bacteria, resulting in a destructive host response and lung infection.[39]

In VAP, placement of the endotracheal tube through the trachea into the lower airway bypasses barriers to aspiration such as the glottis and larynx. Seeding of oropharyngeal organisms into the trachea may occur during passage of the tube. Also, bacteria likely adhere to the endotracheal tube surface, with resulting growth of a bacterial biofilm that seeds detached bacteria into the lower airway. Bacteria in biofilms are resistant to host defenses and antibiotics.[40] The biofilm can also become dislodged and embolize distally to set up foci of infection. The endotracheal tube itself may facilitate infection, acting as a conduit that bypasses the mucociliary "blanket", and pooling of secretions around the cuff of the tube can provide an incubator for pathogenic bacteria.

The oral cavity is an important reservoir of infection for VAP in mechanically ventilated, intensive care unit (MV-ICU) patients.[4] The mouth of the ICU patient becomes colonized by potential respiratory pathogens (PRPs) such as coagulase-positive *Staphylococcus aureus, Pseudomonas aeruginosa,* and enteric species. It has been recommended that efforts should focus on preventing or minimizing respiratory pathogen oral colonization, and by limiting aspiration, antibiotic exposure, and use of invasive devices. Based on several published clinical trials, intra-oral disinfection using oral topical chlorhexidine gluconate (CHX) shows promise as a strategy to reduce potential respiratory pathogen colonization in high-risk subjects, especially VAP in MV-ICU patients (**Table 2**).

The application of oral antiseptic agents such as CHX to reduce the risk of VAP remains controversial despite several randomized clinical trials that evaluated various concentrations of CHX to reduce VAP. The 1996 study by DeRiso reported that pre- and postoperative application of 0.12% CHX reduced nosocomial infections in patients undergoing cardiac surgery but not VAP.[41] In contrast, a randomized, controlled trial showed that 0.2% CHX gel applied only to the teeth and gingival tissues of 228 dentate subjects did not reduce VAP in ICU patients, most of whom had contaminated lungs at study entry.[51] However, possible confounding in this trial included the patient population, type of application (gel), site of application (only teeth and gingiva), primary end points and their definitions, and early stopping based on an estimated infection rate of 30% when the actual rate was 18%. Another study conducted in India investigated 0.2% CHX and found no significant difference in VAP compared with placebo.[48]

A randomized, double-blind, placebo-controlled clinical pilot trial sought to determine the minimal frequency (once or twice a day) for oral decontamination with 0.12% CHX to improve oral hygiene and reduce oral colonization by potential respiratory pathogens in 175 MV patients admitted to the trauma ICU.[49] The primary outcome was quantitative measure of colonization of the oral cavity by target respiratory pathogens. Results showed that neither 0.12% CHX once a day or twice a day showed a significant reduction in dental plaque scores when compared with the placebo. CHX reduced the number of S aureus in dental plaque, but did not reduce the total number of potential respiratory pathogens, or the numbers of enterics, Pseudomonas, or Acinetobacter in the ventilated subjects. A nonsignificant reduction in VAP rate was noted in groups treated with CHX compared with the placebo group ($P = .1459$).

On the other hand, a randomized controlled trial (RCT) conducted by Koeman and colleagues in the Netherlands in five hospitals with mixed ICUs reported that 2.0% CHX in Vaseline applied to the buccal mucosa four times a day significantly reduced VAP compared with placebo.

Several systematic reviews and meta-analyses have been published in the past few years regarding the efficacy of oral CHX or oral decontamination in prevention of pneumonia.[52–56] The general conclusion from these reviews is that topical chlorhexidine for oral care may lead to delayed onset of VAP. There is a need for more evidence, however, because of the heterogeneity of published studies and possible publication bias.

SUMMARY

Much progress has been made in the past decade to determine the impact of periodontal diseases on various systemic diseases. In some cases (adverse pregnancy outcomes, pneumonia, and diabetes) several randomized trials have been conducted to illuminate the potential role for periodontal or oral interventions in prevention of the disease. However, the role of periodontal therapy in the prevention or reduction of these systemic diseases has not been proven by these trials, perhaps because of the limitations of the studies. In some of these cases (diabetes), randomized trials with improved study designs are under way. For other systemic diseases such as CVD, various challenges such as the required long duration of follow-up continue to prevent the conduction of definitive trials. Additional research will be required to understand the value of oral interventions in the prevention of systemic diseases.

REFERENCES

1. Bobetsis YA, Barros SP, Offenbacher S. Exploring the relationship between periodontal disease and pregnancy complications. J Am Dent Assoc 2006; 137(Suppl):7S–13S.
2. Dasanayake AP, Gennaro S, Hendricks-Munoz KD, et al. Maternal periodontal disease, pregnancy, and neonatal outcomes. MCN Am J Matern Child Nurs 2008;33:45–9.
3. Kinane D, Bouchard P. Periodontal diseases and health: consensus report of the Sixth European Workshop on Periodontology. J Clin Periodontol 2008;35(8 Suppl):333–7.
4. Paju S, Scannapieco FA. Oral biofilms, periodontitis, and pulmonary infections. Oral Dis 2007;13:508–12.

5. Kamer AR, Craig RG, Dasanayake AP, et al. Inflammation and Alzheimer's disease: possible role of periodontal diseases. Alzheimers Dement 2008;4: 242–50.
6. Gibson FC 3rd, Yumoto H, Takahashi Y, et al. Innate immune signaling and *Porphyromonas gingivalis*-accelerated atherosclerosis. J Dent Res 2006;85:106–21.
7. Ide M, McPartlin D, Coward PY, et al. Effect of treatment of chronic periodontitis on levels of serum markers of acute-phase inflammatory and vascular responses. J Clin Periodontol 2003;30:334–40.
8. D'Aiuto F, Parkar M, Andreou G, et al. Periodontitis and systemic inflammation: control of the local infection is associated with a reduction in serum inflammatory markers. J Dent Res 2004;83:156–60.
9. Mercanoglu F, Oflaz H, Oz O, et al. Endothelial dysfunction in patients with chronic periodontitis and its improvement after initial periodontal therapy. J Periodontol 2004;75:1694–700.
10. D'Aiuto F, Nibali L, Parkar M, et al. Short-term effects of intensive periodontal therapy on serum inflammatory markers and cholesterol. J Dent Res 2005;84:269–73.
11. Seinost G, Wimmer G, Skerget M, et al. Periodontal treatment improves endothelial dysfunction in patients with severe periodontitis. Am Heart J 2005;149:1050–4.
12. Tonetti MS, D'Aiuto F, Nibali L, et al. Treatment of periodontitis and endothelial function. N Engl J Med 2007;356:911–20.
13. Offenbacher S, Beck JD, Moss K, et al. Results from the Periodontitis and Vascular Events (PAVE) Study: a pilot multicentered, randomized, controlled trial to study effects of periodontal therapy in a secondary prevention model of cardiovascular disease. J Periodontol 2009;80:190–201.
14. Vergnes JN, Sixou M. Preterm low birth weight and maternal periodontal status: a meta-analysis. Am J Obstet Gynecol 2007;196:135. e1–7.
15. Rajapakse PS, Nagarathne M, Chandrasekra KB, et al. Periodontal disease and prematurity among non-smoking Sri Lankan women. J Dent Res 2005;84:274–7.
16. Lopez NJ, Smith PC, Gutierrez J. Periodontal therapy may reduce the risk of preterm low birth weight in women with periodontal disease: a randomized controlled trial. J Periodontol 2002;73:911–24.
17. Lopez NJ, Smith PC, Gutierrez J. Higher risk of preterm birth and low birth weight in women with periodontal disease. J Dent Res 2002;81:58–63.
18. Lopez R. Periodontal treatment in pregnant women improves periodontal disease but does not alter rates of preterm birth. Evid Based Dent 2007;8:38.
19. Michalowicz BS, Hodges JS, DiAngelis AJ, et al. Treatment of periodontal disease and the risk of preterm birth. N Engl J Med 2006;355:1885–94.
20. Offenbacher S, Beck JD, Jared HL, et al. Effects of periodontal therapy on rate of preterm delivery: a randomized controlled trial. Obstet Gynecol 2009;114: 551–9.
21. Jeffcoat MK, Hauth JC, Geurs NC, et al. Periodontal disease and preterm birth: results of a pilot intervention study. J Periodontol 2003;74:1214–8.
22. Polyzos NP, Polyzos IP, Mauri D, et al. Effect of periodontal disease treatment during pregnancy on preterm birth incidence: a metaanalysis of randomized trials. Am J Obstet Gynecol 2009;200:225–32.
23. Wild S, Roglic G, Green A, et al. Global prevalence of diabetes: estimates for the year 2000 and projections for 2030. Diabetes Care 2004;27:1047–53.
24. Mealey BL, Oates TW. Diabetes mellitus and periodontal diseases. J Periodontol 2006;77:1289–303.
25. Taylor GW. Bidirectional interrelationships between diabetes and periodontal diseases: an epidemiologic perspective. Ann Periodontol 2001;6:99–112.

26. Promsudthi A, Pimapansri S, Deerochanawong C, et al. The effect of periodontal therapy on uncontrolled type 2 diabetes mellitus in older subjects. Oral Dis 2005; 11:293–8.
27. Aldridge JP, Lester V, Watts TL, et al. Single-blind studies of the effects of improved periodontal health on metabolic control in type 1 diabetes mellitus. J Clin Periodontol 1995;22:271–5.
28. Jones JA, Miller DR, Wehler CJ, et al. Does periodontal care improve glycemic control? The Department of Veterans Affairs Dental Diabetes Study. J Clin Periodontol 2007;34:46–52.
29. Kiran M, Arpak N, Unsal E, et al. The effect of improved periodontal health on metabolic control in type 2 diabetes mellitus. J Clin Periodontol 2005;32:266–72.
30. Stewart JE, Wager KA, Friedlander AH, et al. The effect of periodontal treatment on glycemic control in patients with type 2 diabetes mellitus. J Clin Periodontol 2001;28:306–10.
31. Darre L, Vergnes JN, Gourdy P, et al. Efficacy of periodontal treatment on glycaemic control in diabetic patients: a meta-analysis of interventional studies. Diabete Metab 2008;34:497–506.
32. Vergnes JN, Arrive E, Gourdy P, et al. Periodontal treatment to improve glycaemic control in diabetic patients: study protocol of the randomized, controlled DIAPERIO trial. Trials 2009;10:65.
33. Novak KF, Taylor GW, Dawson DR, et al. Periodontitis and gestational diabetes mellitus: exploring the link in NHANES III. J Public Health Dent 2006; 66:163–8.
34. Xiong X, Buekens P, Vastardis S, et al. Periodontal disease and gestational diabetes mellitus. Am J Obstet Gynecol 2006;195:1086–9.
35. Xiong X, Elkind-Hirsh K, Vastardis S, et al. Periodontal disease is associated with gestational diabetes: a case-control study. J Periodontology 2009;80:1742–9.
36. Dasanayake AP, Rajapakse S, Jayashankar S, et al. Gum disease as a potential risk factor for gestational diabetes. 5th International Symposium on Diabetes and Pregnancy. Sorrento (Italy), March 26–28, 2009.
37. Flanders SA, Collard HR, Saint S. Nosocomial pneumonia: state of the science. Am J Infect Control 2006;34:84–93.
38. Bonten MJ, Kollef MH, Hall JB. Risk factors for ventilator-associated pneumonia: from epidemiology to patient management. Clin Infect Dis 2004;38: 1141–9.
39. Raghavendran K, Mylotte JM, Scannapieco FA. Nursing home-associated pneumonia, hospital-acquired pneumonia and ventilator-associated pneumonia: the contribution of dental biofilms and periodontal inflammation. Periodontol 2000 2007;44:164–77.
40. Lewis K. Multidrug tolerance of biofilms and persister cells. Curr Top Microbiol Immunol 2008;322:107–31.
41. DeRiso AJ 2nd, Ladowski JS, Dillon TA, et al. Chlorhexidine gluconate 0.12% oral rinse reduces the incidence of total nosocomial respiratory infection and nonprophylactic systemic antibiotic use in patients undergoing heart surgery. Chest 1996;109:1556–61.
42. Genuit T, Bochicchio G, Napolitano LM, et al. Prophylactic chlorhexidine oral rinse decreases ventilator-associated pneumonia in surgical ICU patients. Surg Infect (Larchmt) 2001;2:5–18.
43. Houston S, Hougland P, Anderson JJ, et al. Effectiveness of 0.12% chlorhexidine gluconate oral rinse in reducing prevalence of nosocomial pneumonia in patients undergoing heart surgery. Am J Crit Care 2002;11:567–70.

44. Koeman M, van der Ven AJ, Hak E, et al. Oral decontamination with chlorhexidine reduces the incidence of ventilator-associated pneumonia. Am J Respir Crit Care Med 2006;173:1348–55.

45. Segers P, Speekenbrink RG, Ubbink DT, et al. Prevention of nosocomial infection in cardiac surgery by decontamination of the nasopharynx and oropharynx with chlorhexidine gluconate: a randomized controlled trial. JAMA 2006;296:2460–6.

46. Tantipong H, Morkchareonpong C, Jaiyindee S, et al. Randomized controlled trial and meta-analysis of oral decontamination with 2% chlorhexidine solution for the prevention of ventilator-associated pneumonia. Infect Control Hosp Epidemiol 2008;29:131–6.

47. Bellissimo-Rodrigues F, Bellissimo-Rodrigues WT, Viana JM, et al. Effectiveness of oral rinse with chlorhexidine in preventing nosocomial respiratory tract infections among intensive care unit patients. Infect Control Hosp Epidemiol 2009; 30:952–8.

48. Panchabhai TS, Dangayach NS, Krishnan A, et al. Oropharyngeal cleansing with 0.2% chlorhexidine for prevention of nosocomial pneumonia in critically ill patients: an open-label randomized trial with 0.01% potassium permanganate as control. Chest 2009;135:1150–6.

49. Scannapieco FA, Yu J, Raghavendran K, et al. A randomized trial of chlorhexidine gluconate on oral bacterial pathogens in mechanically ventilated patients. Crit Care 2009;13(4):R117.

50. Munro CL, Grap MJ, Jones DJ, et al. Chlorhexidine, toothbrushing, and preventing ventilator-associated pneumonia in critically ill adults. Am J Crit Care 2009;18: 428–37 [quiz: 38].

51. Fourrier F, Dubois D, Pronnier P, et al. Effect of gingival and dental plaque antiseptic decontamination on nosocomial infections acquired in the intensive care unit: a double-blind placebo-controlled multicenter study. Crit Care Med 2005; 33:1728–35.

52. Pineda LA, Saliba RG, El Solh AA. Effect of oral decontamination with chlorhexidine on the incidence of nosocomial pneumonia: a meta-analysis. Crit Care 2006;10:R35.

53. Kollef MH. Prevention of hospital-associated pneumonia and ventilator-associated pneumonia. Crit Care Med 2004;32:1396–405.

54. Safdar N, Crnich CJ, Maki DG. The pathogenesis of ventilator-associated pneumonia: its relevance to developing effective strategies for prevention. Respir Care 2005;50:725–39.

55. Munro CL, Grap MJ. Oral health and care in the intensive care unit: state of the science. Am J Crit Care 2004;13:25–33.

56. Gastmeier P, Geffers C. Prevention of ventilator-associated pneumonia: analysis of studies published since 2004. J Hosp Infect 2007;67:1–8.

Index

Note: Page numbers of article titles are in **boldface** type.

Moving?

Make sure your subscription moves with you!

To notify us of your new address, find your **Clinics Account Number** (located on your mailing label above your name), and contact customer service at:

Email: journalscustomerservice-usa@elsevier.com

800-654-2452 (subscribers in the U.S. & Canada)
314-447-8871 (subscribers outside of the U.S. & Canada)

Fax number: 314-447-8029

Elsevier Health Sciences Division
Subscription Customer Service
3251 Riverport Lane
Maryland Heights, MO 63043

ELSEVIER

*To ensure uninterrupted delivery of your subscription, please notify us at least 4 weeks in advance of move.

Printed and bound by CPI Group (UK) Ltd, Croydon, CR0 4YY

03/10/2024

01040463-0016